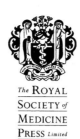

The ROYAL
SOCIETY of
MEDICINE
PRESS Limited

Mental Health in Older People

in Practice

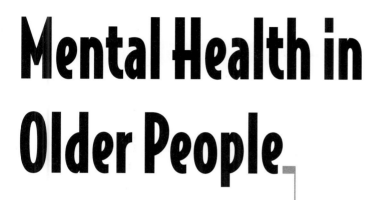

Alistair Burns
Professor of Old-Age Psychiatry,
University of Manchester Department of
Psychiatry Wythenshawe Hospital,
Manchester, UK

Nitin Purandare
Senior Lecturer in Old-Age Psychiatry,
University of Manchester Department of
Psychiatry Wythenshawe Hospital,
Manchester, UK

Sarah Craig
Consultant in Old-Age Psychiatry,
Royal Bolton Hospital NHS Trust, Bolton, UK

©2002 Royal Society of Medicine Press Limited

1 Wimpole Street, London W1G 0AE, UK
207 E Westminster Road, Lake Forest, IL 60045, USA
http://www.rsm.ac.uk

British Library Cataloguing in Publication Data
A catalogue record for this book is available from the British Library

ISBN 1-85315-515-2
ISSN 1473-6845

Phototypeset by Phoenix Photosetting, Chatham, Kent
Printed in Europe by the Alden Group, Oxford

About the authors

Alistair Burns MD FRCP FRCPsych is Professor of Old-Age Psychiatry at the University of Manchester, UK. Professor Burns is Editor-in-Chief of the *International Journal of Geriatric Psychiatry* and is President of the International Psychogeriatric Association. He is also a Non-Executive Director of the South Manchester University Hospitals NHS Trust and Head of the School of Psychiatry and Behavioural Sciences at the University of Manchester. He is a co-author of many books on old-age psychiatry.

Nitin Purandare MBBS DPM DGM MD MRCPsych is a Senior Lecturer in Old-Age Psychiatry at the University of Manchester, UK. He trained in psychiatry in India before completing his specialist training in adult-general psychiatry and old-age psychiatry in Manchester.

Sarah Craig MB MSc MRCPsych is a Consultant in Old-Age Psychiatry at the Royal Bolton Hospitals NHS Trust, Bolton, UK. She trained in general practice before specializing in the field of old-age psychiatry.

Preface

Mental health problems affecting older people are common and adversely affect the person's quality of life. Contrary to general opinion, such problems are not an inevitable consequence of ageing and are eminently treatable. Mental health problems can arise in a number of different settings – an elderly person living at home, someone in a nursing or residential home or, arguably most importantly, when a person is being treated in a general hospital for a medical or surgical illness. Although the cause of the mental health problem can vary, its expression and treatment is likely to be similar in whatever situation it arises.

We have attempted to capture the general principles of presentation and management of various mental health disorders in this short book which is aimed at non-specialists, some of whom may come across an older person with a mental health problem in their daily work, but for whom it is not a consistent or regular event. When formulating a management plan, one cannot better the broad principles of taking a careful patient history, obtaining details from an informant (eg a carer), taking account of the person's physical health and appreciating the individuality of the person's environment. Drugs play a significant part in the treatment of older people with mental health problems; however,

they are by no means the only avenue open to the careful clinician. Not infrequently, symptoms can be short-lived and may be related to changes in a person's physical health or environment. An understanding of such alterations in the patient's life is always helpful when dealing with the situation.

A major problem is the failure to identify mental health problems. Raising awareness of the various forms of dementia and depression, and understanding the implications associated with them could go a long way to correcting this problem. It is also important that clinicians are aware that most of these disorders are amenable to treatment.

We hope that this contribution will be of use to anyone who reads it, whatever their background – medical, nursing, occupational therapy, physiotherapy, speech and language therapy and any of the other professions allied to medicine or social work. It will be a surprise if anyone enjoys reading it more than we have enjoyed writing it.

Alistair Burns
Nitin Purandare
Sarah Craig

May 2002

Acknowledgements

We are indebted to Barbara Dignan whose hard work and editorial skills have made this work possible. We are also grateful to Natalie Baderman and Peter Altman of the RSM Press and Colette Holden for guidance through the project.

Contents

1. Elderly people and their needs

The increasing older population
Social and healthcare impacts

The increasing older population

The UK population aged over 65 years has increased steadily from 5% to 16% of the total population over the past 100 years, and it is predicted that just over one-quarter (about 17 million people) of the whole population will be aged over 60 years by the year 2041 (Table 1.1). This rise is partly due to an average increase in lifespan between 1961 and 2001 of 1.8 years for men and 2.5 years for women (Table 1.2).

> About 25% of the UK population will be aged >60 years in 2041

Table 1.1
UK population 1985–2041

Age (years)	Predicted population (millions)			
	1985	2001	2021	2041
60+	11.8	12.0	14.5	15.4
85+	0.7	1.1	1.3	1.7

Table 1.2
Expectation of life at birth

Year of birth	Life expectancy (years)	
	Males	Females
1841	39	42
1881	47	52
1901	51	58
1921	61	68
1941	69.6	75.4
1961	73.6	79.1
1981	75.5	80.4
1991	76.0	80.8

This population growth is even more marked in developing countries. The increases are dramatic and planning for the economic consequences should be a priority for both healthcare agencies and social care agencies (Table 1.3).

> Dramatic population growth in developing countries should be a priority for healthcare agencies

Table 1.3
Increase in population in developing countries 1975–2000

Age (years)	Increase in population (%)
65–74	33.2
75–79	53.4
80+	64.7

Social and healthcare impacts

Demands on both healthcare and social services provision will grow as a result of the needs of older people:

- 9% of people aged over 60 years encounter severe problems in at least one daily activity
- 80% of people aged over 85 years have some degree of disability, eg vision or hearing impairment
- 50% of people aged over 75 years need home visits by a GP
- 50% of elderly people are looked after at home by informal carers
- 10% of elderly people are dependent entirely on statutory care.

Older people, particularly those over the age of 85 years, tend to be more severely disabled than the younger population. Family support constitutes the main source of care given to older people, with less than half receiving statutory services and less than 10% being entirely dependent on the statutory services. With less than 5% of people in long-term care in the UK, and the government policy of maintaining people in their own homes where possible, pressure on social services is likely to continue. Government documents, such as the White Paper Caring for People, The National Health Service and Community Care Act 1990 and the Carers (Recognition of Services) Act 1995, all underscore the emphasis on community care of elderly people.

The demands on general practice are significant. Table 1.4 shows the impact of these demands on an average-sized general practice.

Table 1.4
The average general practice

Number of patients registered	2000
Number of patients	
Aged 65 years	300
Aged 65–74 years	180
Aged 75+ years	120
Consultation rate/year	
Patients aged 65 years	5823
Patients aged 65–74 years	2607
Patients aged 75+ years	3216
Patients requiring a home visit during 1 year (%)	
Patients aged 65–74 years	20
Patients aged 75+ years	47
Number of patients with dementia	30
Number of patients with functional disorders	93
Affective	78
Psychotic	6
Other, eg hypochondriasis, personality problems	9

Further reading

Godber C, Higgins J. Care for the infirm elderly. A widening of the gap between the poor and better off. *BMJ* 1990; **300**: 555–6.

Hall RG, Channing DM. Age, pattern of consultation and functional disability in elderly patients in one practice. *BMJ* 1990; **301**: 424–8.

Kay DW, Beamish P, Roth M. Old age mental disorders in Newcastle upon Tyne. *Br J Psychiatry* 1964; **110**: 146–58.

Kramer M. The rising pandemic of mental disorders and associated chronic diseases and disabilities. *Acta Psychiatr Scand* 1980; **62(suppl 285)**: 383–96.

Office of Population Censuses and Surveys. *The general household survey*. London: HMSO, 1987.

Office of Population Censuses and Surveys. *Population projections 1985–2025*. London: HMSO, 1987.

Office of Population Censuses and Surveys. *The prevalence of disability among adults*. London: HMSO, 1988.

Post F. The management and nature of depressive illness in late life: a follow through study. *Br J Psychiatry* 1972; **121**: 393–404.

Royal College of General Practitioners Office of Population Censuses and Surveys and Department of Health and Social Security. *Morbidity statistics from general practice 1981–2: third national study*. London: HMSO, 1986.

Williams I. *Caring for older people in the community, 3rd edn*. Oxford: Radcliffe Medical Press, 1995.

2. Mental health disorders

Depression
Psychotic disorders
Dementia
Delirium
Age-related cognitive decline
Anxiety disorders

Depression
Clinical presentation

Sadly, although depression is common in elderly people, it is underdetected and undertreated. Signs and symptoms to look out for include:

- subjective depressive symptoms, eg sadness, loss of interest or enjoyment in normal activities
- biological depressive symptoms, eg early morning insomnia and reduced appetite (in the absence of prominent subjective depressive symptoms)
- deliberate self-harm or overdose
- irritability or agitation
- self-neglect
- marked anxiety about health and wellbeing of themself and relatives
- forgetfulness (dementia-like picture in severe cases)
- multiple physical complaints or physical disability out of proportion to actual impairment
- noncompliance with treatment of physical illness
- recovery or rehabilitation from physical illness that is slower than expected
- overdependence on relatives and carers
- increased alcohol intake

- psychotic symptoms, eg hallucinations and delusions of having serious physical illness or poverty; excessive guilt about trivial mistakes from the past.

> Depression is common in elderly people, but it is underdiagnosed and undertreated

It is not uncommon for a patient to present with depression despite not complaining of a depressed mood. Normally, a depressed patient will present with a preoccupation with physical symptoms. This usually prompts a detailed search for disease, which can reinforce the patient's negative beliefs. Pain can prompt injudicious surgical procedures. Eventually, large numbers of normal investigations convince everyone (except the patient) that the primary problem is not physical illness. Memory complaints can lead to an erroneous diagnosis of dementia.

> Depressed patients often present with physical rather than depressive symptoms

Prevalence

Rates of depressive illness in older people vary between 1 and 3%, but 10–15% of older people have depressive symptoms. Women are usually more affected than men, but in contrast to many other disorders there is no obvious age-related increase in prevalence. Indeed, nonagenarians have lower rates of depression than people in their 60s and 70s. Older people who are in residential care or acute or rehabilitation medical wards have much higher rates of depression (40% in residential care patients and up to 65% in medical in-patients). It may be that exclusion of this group of people from community surveys has led to the relative underestimation of depression in older people.

> Up to 65% of older medical in-patients are clinically depressed

Aetiology

Many factors increase the risk of developing depression. Table 2.1 lists some of these risk factors.

Table 2.1
Risk factors for depression

- Recent bereavement, especially of spouse or partner
- Adverse life events, eg being the victim of crime, moving house
- Living alone with poor social support
- Diagnosis of physical illness, eg heart disease, diabetes, cancer
- Physical illness causing pain (eg arthritis), discomfort (eg breathlessness due to cardiac or lung disease) or reduced mobility (eg fracture, stroke)
- Past episode of depression
- Family history of depression
- Impaired vision or hearing
- Alcohol dependence
- Dementia
- Loss of a pet

Adverse life events, such as being the victim of crime, may lead to symptoms of depression being regarded as 'understandable'. Unfortunately, this is sometimes interpreted as meaning that no treatment is needed.

Prognosis

The prognosis of depression in old age is highly variable:

- 25% of sufferers make a complete recovery
- 25% suffer some residual symptoms
- 40% recover but relapse
- 10% have resistant depression.

Management

Mild depressive symptoms can resolve spontaneously or may clear up after the cause is recognized and dealt with. Supportive counselling may be all that is needed; most patients do not need specialist treatment or drugs. If symptoms become more severe, antidepressants are the treatment of choice. However, it is not unknown for a doctor to suggest a prescription for antidepressants and then review the patient a month later to find they are back to normal. The doctor will be pleased at his/her efficiency and skill of diagnosis, only to find that due to an administrative failure the patient has not actually received the drugs.

Mild depression may disappear spontaneously or may be resolved by recognizing and dealing with the cause

---

There are four main groups of antidepressants (see Table 2.2).

Table 2.2
Classes of antidepressants

- Selective serotonin reuptake inhibitors (SSRIs), eg sertraline, paroxetine, fluoxetine, fluvoxamine, citalopram
- Tricyclic antidepressants, eg amitriptyline, dothiepin, imipramine, lofepramine
- Serotonergic and noradrenergic reuptake inhibitors (SNRIs), eg venlafaxine
- Others, eg mirtazapine, trazodone

Selective serotonin reuptake inhibitors

Selective serotonin reuptake inhibitors (SSRIs) are probably as effective as tricyclic antidepressants. They are increasingly becoming the treatment of choice because of their quick onset of action (effects are noticeable within 2 weeks), lack of anticholinergic side-effects (eg sedation, confusion, blurred vision, dryness, urinary retention), lack of cardiac side-effects (eg arrhythmias, heart block), and greater safety in overdose than tricyclic antidepressants. Table 2.3 gives the recommended doses for some SSRIs.

Table 2.3
Recommended doses of SSRIs

Drug	Starting dose (mg/day)	Standard dose (mg/day)	Maximum dose (mg/day)
Paroxetine	10–20	20–40	40
Fluoxetine	10–20	20–40	40
Sertraline	50	50–100	150
Citalopram	20	20–40	40

SSRIs have a more rapid rate of onset, have fewer anticholinergic and cardiac side-effects, and are safer in overdose than tricyclic antidepressants

Common side-effects of SSRIs include:

- nausea and vomiting
- headache
- insomnia
- convulsions (in at-risk patients, eg people with a history of epilepsy and/or previous convulsions)
- increased agitation and anxiety (especially with fluoxetine)
- anxiety-like withdrawal symptoms if medication suddenly stopped, especially with paroxetine.

SSRIs are normally taken in the morning as they can cause insomnia

Tricyclic antidepressants

The main disadvantages of the tricyclics are their anticholinergic and cardiac side-effects. Also, they can be fatal in overdose. Their main advantage is that their sedative action can help insomnia and anxiety symptoms. Table 2.4 gives the recommended doses for some common tricyclics.

Serotonergic and noradrenergic reuptake inhibitors

Serotonergic and noradrenergic reuptake inhibitors (SNRIs) act on both serotonergic and noradrenergic receptors. They should be considered if there is no response to an SSRI. The only SNRI in clinical use is venlafaxine (see Table 2.5 for recommended doses).

Other antidepressants

There are some other antidepressants, such as mirtazapine (15 mg at night, increased to a

Table 2.4
Recommended doses of some common tricyclic antidepressant drugs

Drug	Starting dose	Standard dose	Maximum dose
Amitriptyline	25–75 mg/day	75–150 mg/day	150 mg/day (divided or at night)
Dothiepin	50–75 mg at night	75–150 mg at night	150 mg at night
Lofepramine	70 mg at night	70 mg twice daily or 140 mg at night	210 mg/day

Table 2.5
Recommended doses for venlafaxine

Starting dose (mg/day)	Standard dose	Maximum dose (mg/day)
37.5, increased to 75 after 3–4 days	75 mg twice daily or 150 mg/day modified release	300

maximum of 45 mg at night) and trazodone (100–300 mg/day), that are also useful, especially if sedation is desired. Monoamine oxidase inhibitors (MAOIs), such as phenelzine and tranylcypromine, may be prescribed by specialist services, but hypertensive reactions can occur as a result of ingestion of tyramine (eg in cheese or red wine) during MAOI use. A washout period of at least 1–2 weeks is required when changing from MAOIs to another antidepressant (especially SSRIs) to avoid serotonergic syndrome. This syndrome is characterized by confusion, restlessness, tremor and sweating often and is seen with concomitant use of SSRIs and MAOIs.

Mood stabilizers

Mood stabilizers are the treatment of choice for the maintenance prophylaxis of manic and depressive illness, but they can also be used in the treatment of mania and resistant depression, and in the control of impulsive behaviour.

Lithium is probably the most common mood stabilizer. The usual dose is 200–600 mg/day, which can be adjusted to maintain blood levels at 0.4–0.8 mmol/l. The side-effects of lithium include:

- gastrointestinal disturbances
- fine tremor
- polyuria
- polydipsia
- weight gain.

Signs of toxicity include coarse tremor, ataxia, nystagmus, dysarthria, renal impairment and convulsions. Lithium should normally be prescribed only following specialist advice.

> Lithium is the most commonly prescribed mood stabilizer

Carbamazepine can be prescribed if lithium is ineffective or not tolerated, if there is renal

impairment, or if there are rapid mood swings (four or more affective episodes per year). The usual dose is 400–600 mg/day in two divided doses, aiming for blood levels of 4–12 mg/l. Contraindications for carbamazepine are:

- atrioventricular conduction defects on electrocardiogram (ECG)
- evidence of bone marrow suppression
- porphyria.

The carbamazepine level should be checked and a full blood count (FBC), liver function tests (LFTs) and renal function tests carried out every 3 months. Side-effects of carbamazepine include nausea, vomiting, ataxia, drowsiness, blurred vision, confusion and rash.

Sodium valproate is an alternative mood stabilizer; the recommended dose is 600–1200 mg/day in two divided doses. Side-effects include gastric irritation, tremor, ataxia, drowsiness and weight gain. Monitoring the levels of sodium valproate in the blood is not very useful because there is no good correlation between blood level and clinical symptoms. However, it is important to carry out regular LFTs and FBCs because sodium valproate can cause liver dysfunction and blood disorders.

Choice of antidepressant

The adage of 'start low, go slow' should be followed. Patients with cardiovascular problems (especially postural hypotension and cardiac arrhythmias) should be tried on an SSRI first. If the patient does not respond despite an adequate therapeutic dose given for at least 6 weeks, then consider adding a second antidepressant (such as an SSRI to a tricyclic, or vice versa) or lithium. If compliance has been poor because of side-effects, then an alternative drug from the same class could be tried. There is good evidence that drugs are effective in patients with coexisting depression and dementia and in those patients with physical illness and depression.

If side-effects have led to poor compliance, try the patient on another drug from the same class of antidepressants

The optimal duration of treatment with antidepressants has yet to be established. However, it has been suggested that continuous treatment for 2 years is associated with a doubled reduction of the relapse rate.

Other treatments

Electroconvulsive therapy (ECT) is well tolerated in older patients and is often regarded as the treatment of choice for patients with delusional depression. Patients with more endogenous features of depression (eg delusions, vegetative symptoms, worthlessness, loss of interest or guilt) respond best. ECT can be used safely in patients with a combination of dementia and depression.

Electroconvulsive therapy is the non-drug therapy of choice for elderly patients with delusional depression

Psychosocial treatments should not be underestimated or ignored when treating elderly people. Precipitating or maintaining factors in their depression for which something can be done, such as social isolation or poor-quality accommodation, should be identified and dealt with wherever possible. Formal support groups, cognitive therapy, family therapy and individual psychotherapy can all be beneficial, but they should be regarded as adjuncts to, rather than replacements of, antidepressant therapy. Bereavement counselling is appropriate if the patient has suffered a loss. It is important to pay attention to the person's social environment, ensuring that social isolation, adequate housing, financial problems, dietary issues and appropriate medication are all addressed.

When prescribing for an elderly patient, it is always important to remember that multiple medications, visual problems, problems with dexterity, depression and memory impairment can all lead to poor compliance.

It is important to address any factors that precipitated or may maintain the depressive symptoms

Mania

The majority (90%) of patients with bipolar affective disorder – episodes of both depression and mania – experience their first manic episode before the age of 50 years. An elderly patient having a manic episode can seem more irritable than happy and, because of agitation, may appear confused. When a manic episode occurs for the first time in an elderly person, it is important to consider frontal lobe pathology (tumours or dementia), syphilis and psychosis in the differential diagnosis. Typical antipsychotics (eg haloperidol) can be used to control agitation in the acute phase. Elderly patients are very susceptible to side-effects, so atypical antipsychotics, such as risperidone or olanzapine, may be the preferred drugs.

Elderly patients are more likely than younger patients to become depressed when recovering from a manic episode. When an elderly person is receiving lithium, it is crucial to give appropriate advice about maintaining hydration and stopping the drug in the short term if vomiting or diarrhoea develops. Coarse tremor and ataxia are signs of toxicity. The lithium blood level and renal function should be checked at least every 3 months when the patient is on a stable dose; thyroid function tests (TFTs) should be carried out annually.

Elderly patients are more likely to become depressed after a manic episode than younger patients

Psychotic disorders

Clinical presentation

Psychosis in older people is a heterogeneous group of disorders characterized by falsely held abnormal beliefs (delusions) and hallucinations (usually auditory or visual). It is crucial to distinguish between disorders that appear for the first time in old age and chronic psychiatric conditions (usually schizophrenia) in patients who have grown old. The latter group is often referred to as 'graduates'.

Psychosis occurring for the first time in an elderly person is most often classified as a delusional disorder (previously called late paraphrenia). The patient gradually develops specific persecutory delusions, the theme of which may be simple, eg hostility and/or suspicion against a neighbour, but may become more elaborate (systematized). Sometimes, the symptoms can be the forerunner of dementia, and it may not become apparent until later that the onset of a delusional idea was an indication of the start of the dementing process. It is important to take a careful history to reveal whether memory loss accompanies the delusion.

Patients with psychotic disorders suffer from abnormal beliefs (delusions) and/or hallucinations

Prevalence

These disorders are relatively uncommon, probably affecting about 1% of the elderly population.

Aetiology

The aetiology of psychosis in older people is multifactorial. The conventional picture of an older patient with late delusional disorder is a person who is female, socially isolated, deaf and who never married. There is usually no past psychotic history, but pre-existing 'eccentric' personality traits may have been present. A significant proportion of these patients has brain abnormalities, such as cerebral infarction or haemorrhage.

Management

The mainstay of the management of an elderly person with late paranoid psychosis is to develop a close empathic relationship with the patient; community psychiatric nurses (CPNs) are usually in the best position to carry this out. Antipsychotics can lessen paranoid beliefs, and are usually best given as depot preparations in doses adjusted for the elderly. Rehousing, although often requested, is generally not a useful strategy because persecutory ideas usually reappear.

Patients with chronic mental illness who grow old can be managed in the same way as their younger counterparts, with the obvious caveats that cognitive impairment may supervene and physical ill-health may complicate the clinical picture. The side-effects of medication tend to be more severe in older people. It should not be forgotten that patients with chronic mental illness have the same rights with regard to medical and surgical treatment as anyone else.

Side-effects of antipsychotic drugs tend to be worse in older patients than in their younger counterparts

Antipsychotic medication

Antipsychotics can be divided into conventional antipsychotics (including depot preparations) and atypical antipsychotics. The following should be considered when selecting antipsychotic medication for an older patient:

- All antipsychotics have roughly the same efficacy.

- Choice depends on predominant symptoms (positive, eg hallucinations or delusions, and negative, eg apathy or lack of motivation) and side-effects profile.

- Older people are five to six times more at risk of developing tardive dyskinesia than younger patients.
- Older people are more prone to confusion due to anticholinergic side-effects than younger patients.

Conventional antipsychotics can be divided into high-potency and low-potency drugs. An example of a high-potency antipsychotic is haloperidol (usual dose 1–5 mg/day in two divided doses or all taken at night), which has a lower risk of sedation and cardiac side-effects but a higher risk of extrapyramidal side-effects. These extrapyramidal side-effects include tremor, cognitive rigidity, mask-like facies, akinesia (reduced or slow movements), increased salivation, acute dystonia (involuntary, sudden spasms of muscle groups) and akathisia (increased restlessness, especially in legs). Low-potency drugs, such as chlorpromazine (25 mg two or three times daily) or promazine (25–50 mg two or three times daily), have the advantage of better control of behavioural disturbance due to their sedative properties.

> Low-potency antipsychotics have fewer cardiac side-effects but a higher risk of extrapyramidal side-effects

ECG monitoring is necessary because of the risk of prolonged QTc interval. Thioridazine has been withdrawn because of concerns over cardiac safety.

Common side-effects of conventional antipsychotics include:

- drowsiness
- anticholinergic side-effects
  - dry mouth
  - blurred vision
  - confusion
  - urinary retention
  - constipation.

Antipsychotics can also be given by intramuscular injection (depot preparations), which is useful if compliance with oral medication is a problem. However, intramuscular injections should not be started unless recommended by a specialist. Older people are at increased risk of local complications at the injection site due to reduced muscle mass. Table 2.6 gives the recommended doses for some depot preparations.

The main advantage of atypical antipsychotics is the reduced risk of extrapyramidal side-effects and tardive dyskinesia. Examples of atypical antipsychotics are risperidone (0.5–1 mg twice daily – this has extrapyramidal side-effects at higher doses) and olanzapine (5–10 mg at night – this is more sedative). Clozapine is not commonly used because of the risk of agranulocytosis and postural hypotension and the need for regular blood tests. Other atypical antipsychotics (amisulpride, quetiapine) have yet to be used extensively in older people.

Table 2.6
Recommended doses for depot preparations of antipsychotics

Drug	Test dose (mg)	Usual dose
Fluphenazine decanoate	6.25	12.5–50 mg every 2–3 weeks
Flupentixol decanoate	10	20–40 mg every 2–3 weeks
Haloperidol decanoate	12.5	50–150 mg every 4 weeks
Zuclopenthixol decanoate	50	100–200 mg every 2–3 weeks

Atypical antipsychotics are less likely than typical antipsychotics to cause extrapyramidal side-effects; however, they tend to be more sedative

Dementia
Clinical presentation

Dementia is not a diagnosis, but is a convenient clinical description of a cluster of signs and symptoms. It is just as unacceptable to be satisfied with a diagnosis of dementia as it would be for a physician to diagnose jaundice but explain that further investigations were not necessary. In the same way that liver damage may be the final pathway to causing jaundice, brain damage is the common pathway to causing dementia. Taking the analogy further, cirrhosis of the liver is one of the causes of jaundice in the same way that Alzheimer's disease is one of the causes of dementia; cirrhosis has a number of causes, just as Alzheimer's disease has multiple aetiologies.

The manifestations of the clinical syndrome of dementia can be divided into three symptom complexes: neuropsychological, neuropsychiatric and problems in carrying out activities of daily living.

The neuropsychological element consists of:

- amnesia (loss of memory)
- aphasia (receptive or expressive, the latter being more apparent in conversation and including nominal aphasia, tested by direct questioning of the naming of objects)
- apraxia (inability to carry out tasks such as dressing oneself or using a knife and fork correctly, despite intact sensory and motor nervous systems)
- agnosia (inability to recognize things such as one's own mirror reflection or a family member – this is not the same as forgetting someone's name).

The neuropsychiatric component consists of symptoms such as psychiatric disturbances and behavioural disorders, which are present in a substantial proportion of patients. The most common of these are (approximate frequencies in brackets):

- depression (up to 66%)
- paranoid ideation (30%)
- misidentification (usually based on agnosia; 20%)
- hallucinations (15%)
- aggression (20%)
- wandering (20%).

The most common hallucinations are auditory. Intercurrent delirium or Lewy body dementia (LBD) should be suspected if visual hallucinations are present.

In the later stages of dementia, difficulties in carrying out activities of daily living are

Table 2.7
Questions that should be asked to determine the possibility of dementia

- Does the person forget people's names?
- Does the person forget appointments?
- Does the person forget conversations they have had?
- Does the person forget where they have put things?
- Does the person tend to repeat things?
- Does the person have trouble paying attention?
- Does the person have difficulty cooking a meal or organizing for bills to be paid?
- Does the person have trouble working new pieces of equipment?
- Does the person have more trouble adding things up in their head than they used to?
- Does the crossword take longer to do than it used to?
- Does the person tend to get flustered in new situations?
- Does the person have difficulty in solving everyday problems that they used to do easily, eg would they know what to do if the lights in the house fused?
- Does the person ever get lost walking familiar routes?
- Does the person ever get lost when driving?
- Does the person ever forget what day it is and have to ask somebody?
- Is the person more irritable than they used to be?
- Has the person's personality changed?
- Is the person less easygoing than they used to be?

manifest by obvious problems in dressing, eating and going to the toilet. In the early stages, there may be a failure to wash or dress to the person's usual standard, self-neglect of the diet (leading to weight loss), and neglect of household tasks. The questions listed in Table 2.7 should be asked to assess the possibility of dementia.

> It is particularly important to document any deterioration from a previous level of functioning

Diagnosis and differential diagnosis

The diagnostic process of dementia is a two-stage procedure. The first stage is to establish a diagnosis of dementia; the second stage is to elucidate the cause of the dementia syndrome. The main differential diagnoses of dementia are:

- depression
- delirium
- normal age-associated memory changes
- toxic effects of drugs.

One situation where the diagnosis is problematic is where there has been chronic poor environmental stimulation (eg in the increasingly rare situations in which the person has been institutionalized for a long time, or when the person has significantly impaired eyesight and/or poor hearing).

One of the most challenging diagnostic problems for psychiatrists is differentiating between dementia and depression in elderly people. Underlying this is the ever-present fear of missing a treatable affective disorder in a patient presenting with dementia. Most clinicians will have seen at least one person diagnosed with dementia whose clinical condition has been transformed by antidepressants or ECT. The most important point is not to dismiss a possible diagnosis of depression when classic or even suggestive clinical features are present.

> It is not unknown for a patient to be diagnosed with dementia only for the condition to be transformed by antidepressants or electroconvulsive therapy

The association between drugs and cognitive impairment is simple in that any drug can cause or contribute to cognitive impairment. Drugs particularly associated with cognitive impairment include those that are known to have an effect on the brain, eg antiepileptics, conventional antipsychotics and antiparkinsonians. The general rule is to suspect all drugs and to be particularly wary when comparing the onset of memory problems with any prescriptions being taken at that time.

> Drugs known to have an effect on the brain are associated with cognitive impairment, eg antiepileptics, conventional antipsychotics and antiparkinsonians

Aetiology

There are many factors that can cause a dementia syndrome, each of which may contribute to the clinical picture. The presentation of a person with severe vitamin B12 deficiency can mimic that of a dementia syndrome, but the clinical features are not so specific that they can be identified before a low serum vitamin B12 level is discovered. Furthermore, a number of conditions can coexist with dementia. In the case of vitamin B12, poor diet can lead to a low B12 level in the blood in a patient with established Alzheimer's disease. Good practice would suggest that vitamins should be supplemented but one could never imagine that it could reverse cognitive impairment. A patient with undiagnosed normal-pressure hydrocephalus (NPH) might have the characteristic triad of dementia, gait disturbance and incontinence, which might alert the clinician to carry out a computed tomography (CT) scan. This in turn might reveal the condition. In such a case, treatment with a ventriculoperitoneal shunt to divert the flow of cerebrospinal fluid may help the clinical symptoms.

> Vitamin B12 deficiency can mimic the symptoms of dementia syndrome

The principal causes of dementia are:

- Alzheimer's disease (60%)
- vascular dementia (20%)
- Lewy body dementia (15%)
- frontal lobe dementia and other causes (5%).

Differential diagnosis of Alzheimer's disease

The first and most important step is to take a full clinical history. Patients are often able to describe their own symptoms, how they started and how they have developed; but if the patient has a significant degree of memory loss, disorientation or confusion, it may be necessary to take the history almost entirely from a relative or carer. Even if the patient is able to describe his or her symptoms accurately, it is always important to check these details with someone else. Table 2.8 lists the questions that should be asked if dementia is suspected.

Table 2.8
Questions that should be asked if dementia is suspected

- When did the symptoms start?
- What was the first symptom?
- Did the symptoms appear suddenly or gradually?
- Have the symptoms progressed suddenly or gradually?
- Were there any special circumstances around the time the symptoms started?
- Is there anything that has made the symptoms worse or better?
- What is the person's reaction to the symptoms?
- Have other people outside the family noticed anything?

> Even if the patient appears able to describe their symptoms fully, the clinical history should be checked with a relative or carer

Information should be gathered from suitable informants. As well as family members, the family GP should be able to describe the patient's family history, past medical and personal history, premorbid personality, social circumstances and family relationships. Discussion with a reliable informant will usually establish the onset and duration of the presenting problems. Difficulties with memory and changes in personality are universal in cases of dementia. Problems encountered with hobbies, such as following a complicated knitting pattern or playing bridge, may be the first changes noted. Family members may supply evidence of psychotic symptoms, such as hallucinations or delusions.

The first signs of dementia are usually those of memory loss. This can be manifest by the patient:

- repeating questions (which can be particularly stressful and irritating for carers).
- forgetting a hitherto remembered birthday or anniversary.
- needing to be reminded of the day or date.
- forgetting appointments to meet friends or family.

Occasionally, the first signs are even more obvious, such as forgetting the names of grandchildren or even children, getting lost while driving or visiting a strange place, or failing to recognize a family member. It is particularly distressing when a spouse to whom a patient has been married for 50 years is not recognized. Emerging difficulties in normal daily activities are also sometimes seen: failure to work the controls on household appliances may become more obvious when the purchase of a new gadget completely dumbfounds the patient. Changes in personality and general demeanour (coarsening of affect, mild irritability, mild disinhibition) are common, but these are usually apparent only in retrospect and, unless very marked (as in the case of frontal lobe dementia), they are rarely a presenting feature.

The presentation of dementia is different from that of delirium in that, with the exception of dementia caused by stroke, the onset is gradual. Onset is characteristically over weeks or months compared with that of delirium, which is usually within hours or days.

> Dementia appears gradually over weeks or months, while delirium usually appears over hours or days

Alzheimer's disease usually has a very insidious onset, and by the time of diagnosis, changes will usually have been present for at least 1 or 2 years. When asked, relatives will often have difficulty recalling the timing of onset, saying that it started very slowly, may have been put down to the normal effects of ageing, and worsened gradually. Occasionally, a particular incident, such as a sudden change while on holiday in a strange place, can precipitate the

recognition of other signs and symptoms of dementia that are present.

Not uncommonly, the death of a spouse uncovers existing symptoms in a person who until then had been protected by a cognitively intact, but often more physically frail husband or wife. This information, which comes out in the subsequent history, is often only known by a son or daughter.

Knowledge of the course of the illness is important in distinguishing vascular dementia from Alzheimer's disease (see Table 2.9). In patients with vascular dementia, the presentation is usually more sudden and onset can often be timed more accurately. The progression over time often follows a more stepwise decline, with periods of weeks or even months of no obvious worsening followed by a sudden deterioration (often coinciding with a further small stroke). Symptomatology is much the same as in Alzheimer's disease, although aphasia can be more prominent, personality changes less marked and depression more apparent. Catastrophic reactions (extreme tearfulness when faced with failure on cognitive tests) and emotional lability also occur more often. Patients with frontal lobe

Table 2.9
Distinguishing features of Alzheimer's disease and vascular dementia

Feature	Alzheimer's disease	Vascular dementia
Cognitive impairment	Diffuse	Patchy
Onset	Insidious	Abrupt
Decline	Slow	Step-like
Stroke/transient ischaemic attack (TIA)	Uncommon	Common
Insight in to the disability	Lost early	Present until late
Emotional lability	Usually absent	Usually present
Depressive symptoms	Common	Very common
Hallucinations/delusions	Common	Less common at presentation
Vascular risk factors	Absent/minimal	Significant
Slowing on electroencephalgraphy (EEG)	Diffuse/symmetric	Patchy/asymmetric
CT scan	Mainly temporal lobe atrophy, absence of significant vascular changes	Infarcts/diffuse white matter hyperintensities

dementia characteristically present with personality changes, repetitive behaviour and depression.

> The symptoms of Alzheimer's disease are very similar to those seen in vascular dementia

Patients with LBD often present with acute or subacute confusional states, falls, florid visual hallucinations and persecutory ideas, together with parkinsonian features, including sensitivity to antipsychotic medication. However, these defined syndromes are not always clearly differentiated clinically. Often, there is considerable overlap, for example patients with Alzheimer's disease may appear to have prominent aphasia and patients with vascular dementia may have frontal lobe symptoms.

Prevalence

Between 3 and 7% of people over the age of 65 years have moderate or severe dementia. The prevalence of mild dementia varies depending on the population surveyed, but there is an average estimate of between 15 and 20% in people aged over 65 years. The prevalence of dementia increases with age (see Table 2.10) and is thought to double every 5–6 years after the age of 65.

> The prevalence of dementia increases with age. After the age of 65, the prevalence is thought to double every 5 or 6 years

Table 2.10
Age-specific prevalence rates for dementia and Alzheimer's disease in Europe

Age (years)	Dementia (%)	Alzheimer's disease (%)
60–69	2.4	0.3
70–79	9.8	3.2
80–89	34.6	10.8
90–100	66.9	Rate not available

Aetiology of Alzheimer's disease and vascular dementia

In some families with Alzheimer's disease, there is a genetic mutation inherited in an autosomal dominant fashion. Mutations in the amyloid precursor protein gene on chromosome 21, presenilin 1 gene on chromosome 14 and presenilin 2 gene on chromosome 1 have all been documented. Apolipoprotein E4 (apoE4) is known to be associated with a greatly increased risk (20-fold) of Alzheimer's disease in people who are homozygous (ie possess two apoE4 alleles), with a lesser but still significant increase in risk (about five-fold) in people who are heterozygous (ie possess one apoE4 allele).

> Homozygosity for the apoE4 allele increases the risk of Alzheimer's disease 20-fold

A number of environmental factors have been implicated in Alzheimer's disease, including exposure to aluminium and head injury. Exposure to aluminium probably causes an encephalopathy resembling dementia rather than being a discrete cause of Alzheimer's disease. Other factors for which there is some evidence include:

- thyroid disease
- physical inactivity
- use of antiperspirants (probably related to aluminium)
- parental age
- ulnar loop patterns on the hands
- snoring.

Oestrogen is known to be a protective factor. A number of studies using a case-control methodology have demonstrated that women taking oestrogen have a lower rate of Alzheimer's disease compared with those not taking supplementation. There is also evidence to show that patients with Alzheimer's disease who have taken oestrogen have less cognitive impairment and that their disease starts later. Some trials have suggested that oestrogen improves cognitive function in Alzheimer's disease, and there seems to be an added beneficial effect with combined oestrogen and anticholinesterases. Nonsteroidal anti-inflammatory agents have also been described as having a possible protective effect.

The aetiology of vascular dementia is shared with cerebrovascular disease in general, ie genetic predisposition and the environmental risk factors of hypertension, diabetes, smoking and obesity. The causes of LBD and frontal lobe dementia are unknown.

Examination and investigations

Examination of the patient's mental state will show evidence of any self-neglect. Indicators of depression, for example physical illness, disinhibited or inappropriate behaviour, agitation or retardation may be apparent. Guarded or hostile behaviour may indicate underlying paranoid ideas. Poor attention span (indicating clouding of consciousness) may be apparent, and can be helpful in differentiating delirium from dementia.

The patient's speech will reveal any evidence of aphasia or dysarthria. Abnormalities of speech seen in advanced dementia include perseveration (the patient continues to give an answer to the previous question in response to new questions), palilalia (repeating the last word of a question with increasing frequency), logoclonia (repeating the last syllable) and logorrhoea (meaningless outpouring of words). The patient may echo the examiner's speech (echolalia) or actions (echopraxia). The content of thought is often impoverished, but careful questioning will reveal the presence of delusions or depressive ideas, and the patient may reveal psychotic experiences.

Affective symptoms are often found in association with dementia and may be the presenting feature; agitation, anxiety or irritability are pointers to such symptoms. Disorders of perception occur frequently in people with dementia, and features suggestive of visual or auditory hallucinations will be apparent from the history. It is not uncommon for a patient to hallucinate in the presence of the examiner.

In the mental state examination it is important to:

- observe for agitation, retardation or self-neglect
- ask about the symptoms of depression
- enquire about psychotic symptoms
- observe any obvious manifestations of physical illness
- carry out cognitive function tests.

Specific questioning may reveal psychotic symptoms, such as paranoid ideas or misidentifications.

Assessment of cognitive function is aided greatly by using a standard test such as the mini-mental state examination (MMSE, see Chapter 8). The MMSE is scored out of 30 points – 10 of which are given for orientation in time and place, and the remaining 20 for tests of attention, registration, recall, language, manipulating information and praxis. It has been suggested that a cut-off score of 23 or 24 is a satisfactory discriminator between cognitive dysfunction and normality. The MMSE is a useful screening instrument in clinical assessment of patients referred with a possible dementia, but it is not a substitute for a full history and mental state examination. It is quick and easy to complete and sensitive to changes over time, with an expected decline of about three points each year in a patient with Alzheimer's disease.

> The MMSE is a useful test for assessing cognitive function; however, it must not replace taking a full clinical history

A physical examination should be carried out, with specific reference to the central nervous system; high blood pressure and focal neurological signs may indicate vascular disease. Assessment of vision and hearing is important, as impairment of these may exaggerate cognitive decline.

Further investigations should be minimally invasive and relatively cheap. Screening tests are aimed at picking up any reversible cause of a dementia syndrome. However, there is disagreement as to which tests are necessary, and it may be argued that the low number of treatable causes of dementia makes such tests superfluous. A standard screen (see Table 2.11) should include an FBC (for alcoholic dementia), erythrocyte sedimentation rate (ESR), vitamin B12 and folate, urea and electrolytes (U&Es) (for metabolic disorders), calcium and phosphates (for parathyroid disorder), syphilis serology (for general paralysis of the insane), human immunodeficiency virus (HIV) testing where appropriate (for AIDS dementia), chest X-ray and ECG if indicated by abnormalities on clinical examination. Lumbar puncture may be indicated if there is any evidence of encephalitis. CT screening is the radiological investigation of choice to exclude intracranial lesions, while magnetic resonance imaging (MRI) is used for a more detailed assessment of cerebral structure. Single photon emission computed tomography (SPECT) can reveal deficits in blood flow and is helpful in diagnosing frontal lobe and vascular dementia. Electroencephalography (EEG) is sensitive to the confirmation of the diagnosis of delirium.

Guidelines have been published that suggest the circumstances under which a CT scan should be performed. Where the duration of the illness is short (<6 months and certainly <3 months), and where the features of the illness indicate that there may be focal cerebral pathology, the chance of a CT scan detecting a clinically significant lesion is increased. Such features include focal neurological signs, epileptic fits, variations in the course of the illness and indicators of the presence of NPH (gait disturbance and incontinence in the presence of dementia).

Potentially reversible causes of dementia are found in approximately 13% of cases, but only about 1% of patients actually reverse with treatment. However, a higher proportion may show a partial response to treatment. The most common causes of reversible or partially reversible dementia are drugs, depression, thyroid disease, vitamin B12 deficiency, calcium disturbance, liver disease, NPH, subdural haematoma and neoplasm.

Although 13% of dementia cases are caused by reversible factors, only 1% of cases actually reverse after treatment

---

Other dementias
Dementia with Lewy bodies

Lewy body dementia (LBD) is increasingly recognized as a cause of dementia. Specific clinical features are progressive cognitive decline interfering with social or occupational functioning (although memory loss may not be an early feature) and at least one of the following: fluctuating cognition with pronounced variation in attention and alertness, recurrent visual hallucinations and spontaneous motor features of parkinsonism.

Conventional antipsychotics are best avoided in people with LBD as patients can be very sensitive to extrapyramidal side-effects. Anticholinesterases are likely to become useful

---

Table 2.11
Investigations that should be carried out in a person with suspected dementia

- Full blood count (FBC) and erythrocyte sedimentation rate (ESR)
- Blood glucose
- Vitamin B12 and folate
- Thyroid function tests (TFTs)
- Urea & electrolytes (U&E)
- Liver function tests (LFTs)
- Midstream urine sample (MSU)
- Chest X-ray
- Electrocardiogram (ECG)
- Electroencephalography (EEG)
- Computed tomography (CT) scan

alternatives to antipsychotics in these patients, but currently they are not licensed for this use. If psychotic symptoms become prominent, careful use of sedatives (eg clomethiazole) or atypical antipsychotics (eg olanzapine or low-dose risperidone to a maximum of 2 mg/day) may be justified. Anticonvulsants (eg carbamazepine, sodium valproate) have also been found to be useful. Patients can be very distressed and disturbed by their hallucinations, and giving benzodiazepines (eg lorazepam, diazepam) for a short time can be beneficial.

> Typical antipsychotics should be avoided in LBD patients as these people tend to be very sensitive to the extrapyramidal effects of the drugs

Frontotemporal dementia

Frontotemporal dementia (FTD) tends to be more common in women and usually starts in the fifth decade of life. As the name suggests, it predominantly affects the frontal and temporal lobes. Specific features include disinhibition, lack of judgement, social inappropriateness, apathy, lack of concern, stereotypy, mannerisms and hyperorality (eating unusual things or excessive consumption of a particular food). Spatial awareness, orientation to time and activities of daily living may remain intact until the later stages. FTD can be difficult to manage and is very distressing to the carer. A SPECT scan often shows diagnostic changes.

Alcohol-induced dementia

Chronic, heavy use of alcohol can lead to an amnesic syndrome affecting predominantly anterograde memory or new learning. Cognitive functions are also affected in a way resembling dementia. Vitamin supplementation (eg with thiamine) and abstinence from alcohol may arrest the progression or partially reverse the dementia.

Normal-pressure hydrocephalus

Normal-pressure hydrocephalus (NPH) is characterized by a triad of cognitive impairment, unsteady gait and incontinence. It is secondary to obstruction of cerebrospinal fluid flow in the subarachnoid space or failure of its normal absorption. A brain scan will show extreme ventricular dilation out of proportion to brain atrophy. It is desirable to obtain a neurosurgical opinion, as a shunt may stop or slow the progression of the disease.

Creutzfeldt–Jakob disease

Creutzfeldt–Jakob disease (CJD) is rare. It can present as dementia, but the decline is usually rapid, with myoclonus and a characteristic EEG showing triphasic wave activity.

Management
Pharmacological treatments

The rationale for the use of drugs in the treatment of cognitive decline in Alzheimer's disease is that they prevent the breakdown of acetylcholine, one of the main neurotransmitters deficient in the disease, thus raising the level of the neurochemicals in the brain.

Tetrahydroaminoacridine (THA), or tacrine, was the first anticholinesterase to be widely available. Although there were statistically significant improvements over placebo, the tolerability and side-effects limited the usefulness of the drug. About 70% of patients were unable to tolerate the gastrointestinal side-effects coupled with the major consequence of liver transaminitis. Better-tolerated drugs, such as donepezil, rivastigmine and galantamine are now available, making tacrine obsolete.

> The development of new, better-tolerated anticholinesterases has made tacrine, the original anticholinesterase, obsolete

Donepezil was released for marketing in the UK in early 1997 and has probably had the greatest impact so far on the treatment of

Alzheimer's disease. Studies show an improvement in both cognition and global improvement, with a greater effect with 10 mg than with 5 mg. In one of the main studies, 42% of patients on placebo had worse global functioning at the endpoint compared with 20% on donepezil. An improvement of seven points on the ADAS-Cog scale is regarded as being of clinical significance: on this basis, improvement was seen in 8% of patients on placebo, 15% on 5 mg donepezil and 25% on 10 mg donepezil. On the clinician's interview-based impression of change (CIBIC) scale, 11% improved in the placebo group compared with 26% on 5 mg donepezil and 25% on 10 mg donepezil. The most common side-effects of donepezil are gastrointestinal, including nausea, vomiting, diarrhoea and anorexia. Some patients develop muscle cramps, headache, dizziness, syncope or flushing. Haematological side-effects include anaemia and thrombocytopoenia, while cardiac side-effects include bradyarrhythmia, fatigue and agitation.

> Donepezil is associated with gastrointestinal, cardiac and haematological side-effects. Some patients taking the drug also experience headaches, dizziness, syncope, flushing and muscle cramps

Rivastigmine was licensed in the UK 1 year after donepezil. It has an effect on both acetylcholinesterase and butyrylcholinesterase. Rivastigmine has a half-life of 2 hours, but cholinesterase inhibition in the brain is thought to last for up to 10 hours. The main drawbacks of rivastigmine are its short half-life, the consequent twice-daily dosing, and the necessity for slow titration to minimize the cholinergic side-effects. Trial data suggest that side-effects of rivastigmine are no worse than those of donepezil; they include nausea, vomiting and anorexia.

Galantamine, a tertiary alkaloid, is a competitive, reversible inhibitor of acetylcholinesterase; it therefore increases the amount of acetylcholine available in the synaptic cleft. Galantamine also acts as an allosteric modulator of nicotinic acetylcholine receptors in the brain. Like all acetylcholinesterase inhibitors, galantamine has the usual tolerability problems. Unless titrated slowly, the majority of its side-effects are gastrointestinal. Galantamine has a half-life of about 8 hours and thus needs to be administered twice daily; the optimal dose is between 16–24 mg/day.

There is little doubt that the acetylcholinesterase inhibitors are statistically and clinically superior to placebo in improving cognitive deficits, global ratings of dementia and activities of daily living in Alzheimer's disease patients. What is also evident is that higher doses of all of the drugs discussed above are consistently more effective than lower doses. The duration of effect and long-term safety of the drugs has yet to be fully established, but cholinesterase inhibitors are likely to be the cornerstones of pharmacological treatment for cognitive deficits in Alzheimer's disease for the foreseeable future.

> Anticholinesterases are likely to remain the drugs of choice for the treatment of Alzheimer's disease for some time

Table 2.12 shows the daily costs to the NHS of prescribing anticholinesterases.

The National Institute of Clinical Excellence has approved the use of donepezil, rivastigmine and

Table 2.12
Costs to the NHS of anticholinesterase drugs

Drug	Dose (mg/day)	Cost (£)
Donepezil	5	2.44
	10	3.42
Rivastigmine	3–12	2.25
Galantamine	8	1.95
	16	2.44
	24	3.00

galantamine in the treatment of mild to moderate Alzheimer's disease under the following conditions:

- MMSE score >12/30
- specialist diagnosis and assessment
- compliance likely
- treatment initiated by specialists
- review after 2–4 months then every 6 months thereafter
- continue if there is evidence of benefit.

Table 2.13 summarizes the main points made in this section about anticholinesterases.

Table 2.13
Summary of anticholinesterases

- Consider referral of patients with suspected dementia to a specialist clinic
- The GP may be asked to take part in a shared-care protocol
- Anticholinesterases can improve or stabilize symptoms in about two-thirds of patients
- Anticholinesterases offer symptomatic control for up to 2 years and possibly longer
- Anticholinesterases act by inhibiting the enzyme cholinesterase, hence increasing the available acetylcholine. A lack of acetylcholine is thought to be responsible for memory impairment
- Drugs available: donepezil (5–10 mg/day), rivastigmine (1.5–6 mg twice daily), galantamine (8–24 mg/day)
- Common side-effects: nausea, vomiting, diarrhoea, agitation, insomnia and dizziness
- Contraindications: left bundle branch block on ECG

The excitatory neurotransmitter glutamate may also play a role in the pathogenesis of dementia. Glutamate antagonists cause deficits in learning and memory in animals. Memantine, an uncompetitive antagonist at the N-methyl-D-aspartate receptor is currently undergoing evaluation for use in Alzheimer's disease and vascular dementia.

Management of vascular dementia

Management involves control of vascular risk factors, such as smoking, hypertension, diabetes and hypercholesterolaemia. It also includes treatment of noncognitive symptoms, such as depression, and taking aspirin to reduce the risk of vascular insult to the brain. Anticholinesterases are not currently licensed for patients with vascular dementia, but this may change.

Management of neuropsychiatric features of dementia

This is essentially the same for all forms of dementia, regardless of the cause. Antipsychotics are the drugs most commonly used to treat behavioural disorders, and they are regarded as being moderately effective. It is well documented that they improve anxiety and mood, and reduce aggression, agitation, hostility and uncooperativeness. The primary efficacy is similar for all antipsychotics, but their side-effects and induced tolerance are variable. They are certainly effective in treating agitation and restlessness; a number of meta-analyses of the literature have shown that in Alzheimer's disease, about 20% of patients with agitation will benefit from antipsychotics. More recent studies have concentrated on Alzheimer's disease, whereas many earlier studies also included patients with acute confusional states. There are no absolute rules on dosage, but generally a lower dose should be used than might be used in a psychotic patient without cognitive impairment.

The side-effects are probably more marked in patients who have dementia than in other patients. They comprise extrapyramidal signs, tardive dyskinesia (in up to 50% of patients), postural hypotension, sedation (due to blockage of histamine receptors), anticholinergic effects, agranulocytosis, and liver and cardiac toxicity. Antipsychotics can cause higher mortality and morbidity in patients with LBD. When selecting a specific agent, there may be little to choose between the main antipsychotics. As with other drugs, choice is often determined on the basis of familiarity.

The side-effects of antipsychotics tend to be more severe in people with dementia than in nondemented patients

A number of non-antipsychotic drugs are also used in the management of patients with dementia. Antidepressants can control agitation and restlessness, and not necessarily just in patients with obvious depressive features, although they are specifically effective when depression is present. Other antidepressants, such as MAOIs and SSRIs, have been used and may be beneficial. Trazodone seems to be particularly helpful in controlling screaming. Some anticonvulsants are used to control agitation. A few case reports suggest that lithium improves agitation, but because of its relative toxicity and the need for monitoring, it is not likely to become a treatment of first choice.

Buspirone, which is a gamma aminobutyric acid (GABA) antagonist, is said to have some effect on agitated patients. Beta-blockers have traditionally been used to control aggression in younger patients with brain damage. Benzodiazepines should not be forgotten: in cases where there is a clinical suspicion of LBD, a combination of benzodiazepines and chlormethiazole can be effective.

Delirium
Clinical presentation

Delirium (confusional state) is an acute disturbance of brain function (compared with the chronic disturbance of dementia) that begins quickly and in which the primary disorder is one of attention and disorganized thinking. Other features include fluctuation in the clinical features, disturbance in the sleep/wake cycle and the presence of psychiatric disorders – normally hallucinations.

The primary disorders of delirium are disorganized thinking and problems with attention

Prevalence

The prevalence of delirium depends on the population studied. In community samples, it is low because delirium is a condition that often quickly comes to the attention of others, leading to treatment and possibly admission to hospital. Six per cent of people in nursing homes are thought to suffer from delirium, but the rate can rise to 60% in medical and surgical wards.

Up to 60% of patients in medical and surgical wards suffer from delirium

Aetiology

The aetiology of delirium is that of the underlying physical disorder; these are many and varied. Predisposing factors include:

- increasing age
- the presence of dementia
- previous alcohol abuse
- prolonged surgical procedures.

The most common causes in clinical practice are urinary and respiratory infections, heart failure and carcinomatosis. Less common factors are transient ischaemic attack (TIA), various drugs (particularly those with anticholinergic actions, eg amitriptyline, levodopa, chlorpromazine), drug interactions, withdrawal from alcohol or benzodiazepines, metabolic imbalances such as renal or hepatic failure, hypoglycaemia and cerebral anoxia.

Prognosis

Delirium tends to start quickly and have a relatively short duration (almost always less than 4 weeks). Conventional teaching is that delirium lasts longer than is commonly supposed in elderly people, and an illness lasting for many weeks should not exclude a diagnosis of delirium. Dementia and delirium often occur together. The mortality is high and is related to the severity of the underlying physical illness, which underscores the need for accurate diagnosis.

Investigations

Full physical examination should include neurological examination, monitoring of pulse, blood pressure and temperature, and an assessment of the level of consciousness. Physical investigations should include blood tests (FBC, ESR, U&Es, LFTs, TFTs, glucose, vitamin B12, folate), urine culture, chest X-ray and ECG. It is useful to do an ECG as occasionally patients who become acutely paranoid have had a myocardial infarction. A CT scan is indicated if an intracranial lesion is suspected.

Management

The two strands to treatment include discovery and treatment of the underlying cause, and symptomatic control of agitation and psychiatric disturbance. Traditional teaching suggests that patients should be nursed in a well-lit room in isolation. However, these measures may be unnecessary and there are no empirical data to support their use. The drug treatment of choice is haloperidol, but care must be used because of its long half-life and tendency to cause extrapyramidal effects.

> Careful monitoring of a patient taking haloperidol for delirium is important as the drug can cause extrapyramidal side-effects

Age-related cognitive decline

It is known that memory declines with age and this has stimulated a number of descriptions of age-related cognitive decline. Benign senile forgetfulness (BSF) is a nonprogressive, mild memory disorder. A person suffering from BSF will make minor errors with respect to orientation but shows no clinical evidence of a progressive memory problem. Age-associated memory impairment (AAMI) has specific diagnostic criteria:

- age over 50 years
- history of gradual memory dysfunction apparent in activities of daily life
- subjective memory complaints substantiated by objective memory deficits, as measured by a performance at least one standard deviation below the mean established for young adults, on a well-standardized memory test
- intact global intellectual function
- absence of dementia as determined by a score of 24 or higher on the MMSE.

A crucial distinction between these criteria and those of BSF is that they were defined in terms of memory loss that was one standard deviation below that for young adults; this was criticized because of its tendency to include the majority of people over the age of 50 years. The analogy was made between the presence of poor eyesight and poor hearing, and whether these would be regarded as abnormal. Also, no specific tests were proposed, nor was it specified how many tests an individual would have to get a low score on to qualify for such a diagnosis. The crucial issue in AAMI is to exclude any of the competing causes of cognitive impairment and any physical disorder. It may be necessary to assess the patient after 6 or 12 months to assess any deterioration. There is evidence to suggest that the rate of the development of dementia at follow-up is five to 10 times higher than in the normal population.

Anxiety disorders

Generalized anxiety disorder and panic disorder, with or without agoraphobia, are not uncommon in elderly people. It is important to look for underlying depression and to rule out possible organic causes, such as heart disease, thyroid problems and carcinomatosis. Alcohol may be also a contributory cause.

Management

Benzodiazepines, although very effective, should not be used for more than 4 weeks as dependence is possible. Antidepressants are often the first choice of treatment, even in the absence of clinical depression. Anxiety-management groups and cognitive behaviour therapy can have far-reaching effects in the long term. The role of the family, support worker or community nurse is crucial to avoid the elderly person becoming chronically housebound, with lower self-esteem, social isolation and eventual depression.

Further reading

Atkinson R. Late onset problem drinking in older adults. *Int J Geriatr Psychiatry* 1994; **9**: 321–6.

Henderson A, Jorm A, Korten A *et al*. Environmental risk factors for Alzheimer's disease. *Psychol Med* 1992; **22**: 429–36.

Howard R, Almeida O, Levy R. Phenomenology, demography and diagnosis in late paraphrenia. *Psychol Med* 1994; **24**: 397–410.

Jones R. *Drug treatment in dementia*. Oxford: Blackwell Science, 2000.

Kay D. The English language literature on late paraphrenia from 1950. In: Howard R, Rabins P, Castle D (eds). *Late onset schizophrenia*. Petersfield: Wrightson Biomedical Publishing, 1999: 17–43.

Mulligan I, Fairweather S. Delirium – the geriatrician's perspective. In: Jacoby R, Oppenheimer C (eds). *Psychiatry in the elderly, 2nd edn*. Oxford: Oxford University Press, 1997: 507–26.

3. Approach to specific problems

The depressed patient
The suicidal patient
The paranoid patient
The aggressive patient
The confused patient
The mentally ill patient who refuses treatment
The patient found wandering
The person with a positive family history of Alzheimer's disease

There are some common underlying principles to managing patients with depression. It is important to start by taking a detailed history from both the patient and the carer. Then:

- Arrange for any appropriate investigations to help rule out underlying physical problems.
- Consider drugs, particularly drug interactions, as the cause.
- Ask about associated symptoms when a specific diagnosis is suspected.
- Assess the severity of the symptoms and their effects on the patient's daily life.
- Consider any issues relating to the safety of the patient and the carer.
- Do not avoid asking questions relating to suicide.
- Consider the possible stress on the carer.
- Review the patient's past history before selecting specific medication.
- Identify specific services that may be able to help.
- Involve the patient and the carer in decision making.
- Arrange for follow-up.

> Taking a detailed history of the patient is essential

The depressed patient

Depressed patients frequently present with physical symptoms, such as dyspnoea, dizziness or pain, rather than psychological symptoms. As in all specialties, taking a detailed history is crucial in eliciting symptoms. Table 3.1 lists the signs and symptoms that should be documented.

Table 3.1
Signs and symptoms that should be recorded (if present) in a depressed patient

- Sleep disturbances
- Diurnal mood variation, particularly if worse in the morning
- Anxiety symptoms, eg panic attacks, churning in the stomach, palpitations and dizziness
- Impaired appetite
- Weight variation
- Subjective memory loss
- Loss of interest in normal activities
- Social isolation
- Fatigue or loss of energy
- Irritability
- Suicidal ideas
- Self-neglect
- Psychomotor agitation or retardation
- Poor concentration

> Depressed patients often present with physical rather than psychological symptoms

When taking a history, it is important to assess the patient's current mental state, focusing on possible suicidal ideas, feelings of worthlessness or guilt and psychotic ideas such as nihilistic beliefs (eg belief that parts of the body are not working). To help formulate the management plan, an assessment of the patient's insight is important.

If depression is likely, it is important to exclude any physical causes that may be contributing to the illness, such as pain, heart failure or endocrine disorders. A physical examination and routine blood tests [full blood count (FBC), erythrocyte sedimentation rate (ESR), liver and renal profiles, glucose level and thyroid function tests (TFTs)] are recommended.

The patient should be referred to specialist services if any of the following are present:

- suicidal thoughts
- psychotic symptoms, eg delusions of worthlessness, guilt, nihilistic ideas
- unresponsiveness to a course of antidepressants
- reduced fluid and dietary intake
- lack of social support
- past history of depression
- significant family history of depression.

Selective serotonin reuptake inhibitors (SSRIs) should be the first choice of treatment for depression. The antidepressant effects of SSRIs may be evident within the first 2 weeks; if there is only a partial response after 6 weeks, then the dose may have to be increased. If there is no response by 6 weeks, then the patient should either be tried on a drug from another class of antidepressants, eg venlafaxine – a serotonergic and noradrenergic reuptake inhibitor (SNRI), or referred to a specialist service for review of the diagnosis and advice about management. For further details on the treatment of depression, see Chapter 2.

The suicidal patient

If a patient has attempted suicide, it is vital to find out exactly what has happened from both the patient and, if possible, another source. It is important to discover the patient's intention at the time and to assess the risk of future self-harm. At a minimum, the following information should be elicited:

- premeditated planning and preparation involved in the suicide attempt

- presence and content of a suicide note
- any recent alterations of financial affairs
- mode of attempted self-harm
- beliefs about the likely effect of the attempt
- how the patient was discovered
- associated alcohol ingestion
- past history of suicide attempts
- past history of other mental health problems
- social support
- recent bereavement
- coexisting physical illness.

A current mental state examination should be carried out to discover whether the patient is still experiencing suicidal ideas, shows any remorse for the act and, importantly, has any symptoms of mental illness (depression, paranoid psychosis, dementia, alcohol abuse, mania, schizophrenia, anxiety symptoms).

> It is important to find out whether a patient who has attempted suicide has any symptoms of mental illness

Suicidal ideas in elderly patients are associated with a high mortality rate, and advice from specialist psychiatric services should be sought. It may be necessary to transfer the patient to a psychiatric ward, using the Mental Health Act if required.

The paranoid patient

It is important to take a history, although it can be difficult to obtain this directly from the patient, who may have limited insight into his or her problems. An informant is therefore crucial. Typical symptoms of paranoia include:

- persecutory thoughts, eg that neighbours are watching them, talking about them or interfering with their house with the aim of trying to remove them from their home (eg altering the gas supply)

- believing that food and drink are being tampered with
- believing medical or nursing staff are plotting against them
- believing members of their family are conspiring against them
- systemized delusional ideas involving complex beliefs that incorporate several people, eg the idea 'someone is against me' may become 'my neighbour is against me: he was watching me, and he has bugged my house', leading to 'my neighbour is a member of the Labour Party, therefore the government is after me'.

Other information that should be sought includes whether the paranoia is acute or chronic, whether there are associated hallucinations (auditory, visual, somatic or olfactory) or mood disorders, and whether the patient has ideas of harm towards people they think are against them. It is important to assess any ideas of self-harm, history of alcohol or drug abuse, forensic history and premorbid personality.

> It may be difficult to obtain a history from a paranoid patient as they may be unwilling to reveal details about themselves. They may also be suspicious of the interviewer's motives

Management should include a physical examination and routine blood tests to exclude confusional state. Any risk to the patient and other people should be assessed, and admission to a specialist hospital ward should be considered if appropriate.

Oral or depot antipsychotic medication may be used. Atypical antipsychotics, eg risperidone and olanzapine are preferable in elderly patients because they have fewer side-effects. Small doses should be given to begin with, eg haloperidol 0.5 mg twice daily or risperidone 0.5 mg twice daily.

It may be useful to engage a community mental health team, including a community psychiatric nurse and a social worker.

The aggressive patient

When faced with an aggressive patient, it is important to consider the safety of the patient, staff, neighbours and other patients. Table 3.2 lists the possible causes of aggression.

Table 3.2
Causes of aggression

- Acute confusional state
- Alcohol/drug withdrawal or intoxication
- Pain
- Hypoglycaemia
- Dementia (eg vascular dementia, Alzheimer's disease, Lewy body dementia)
- Hypomania or mania
- Paranoid illness

If no information is available about the patient's past history, then baseline investigations should be carried out, including temperature, pulse, blood pressure, physical examination, routine blood tests, chest X-ray, urine sample and electrocardiogram (ECG).

> Consider the safety of everybody involved with an aggressive patient when deciding on an appropriate course of treatment

Skilled nurses should aim to treat the patient in a low-stimulating environment, away from other vulnerable patients and keep the patient hydrated and nourished. Antipsychotic medication can be given, ideally orally but intramuscularly if the patient is very aggressive. Small doses should be used in elderly patients, eg haloperidol 0.5 mg three times daily or lorazepam 0.5 mg three times daily. Clinicians ought to be cautious when using antipsychotics in patients with Lewy body dementia, as such drugs may cause extrapyramidal symptoms.

The confused patient

Acutely confused patients should initially be treated by a physician rather than a psychiatrist, as it is vital to investigate and treat physical causes. The patient must be adequately hydrated and nourished, and where possible, a familiar environment should be maintained (ie avoid changing wards). Try to avoid oversedation; if necessary, give small doses of short-acting benzodiazepines (eg lorazepam 1–2 mg as needed) or antipsychotics (eg haloperidol or risperidone 0.5 mg twice daily).

> It is important to avoid oversedation in confused elderly patients because it could mask physical illness and may make patients prone to decubitus ulcers, chest infections or deep vein thrombosis

The mentally ill patient who refuses treatment

If a patient with suspected or known mental illness refuses investigation or treatment for physical illness, the following questions must be asked:

- What are the reasons for the refusal?
- Is the intervention necessary?
- What are the risks and benefits of alternative interventions?
- Does the patient have the capacity to consider the various options?
- Are there any advance directives in force?
- Will the treatment be covered under common law, ie is it an emergency life-saving procedure?

The Mental Health Act does not cover intervention for physical illness, so it may be necessary to consider seeking a psychiatric opinion.

The patient found wandering

If a person is found wandering, the first thing to do is investigate for causes of delirium and check for underlying dementia, eg take a history of cognitive decline from the carer or carry out a mini-mental status examination (MMSE). Use of mild tranquillizers or hypnotics can be considered if nocturnal confusion is part of the dementia.

Ask the carer to reduce the risk of wandering by implementing simple measures, eg locking the doors of the patient's home. The patient may also benefit from a psychogeriatric assessment.

The person with a positive family history of Alzheimer's disease

If a person is worried about Alzheimer's disease because of a positive family history, first obtain a history from the patient and a relative or carer about cognitive decline. An MMSE should also be carried out and if dementia is suspected, blood investigations should be arranged (see Chapter 2).

It is important to emphasize that only a minority of cases of Alzheimer's disease are hereditary. There is no genetic test to establish the diagnosis: the presence of the apolipoprotein E4 (apoE4) allele only suggests an increased risk. A neuropsychological assessment should be carried out and the patient reviewed 1 year later. It might be useful to refer the patient to specialist services that offer genetic counselling and a memory clinic.

> Presence of the apoE4 allele suggests an increased risk for Alzheimer's disease, but it is not diagnostic

Further reading

Folstein MF, Folstein SE, McHugh PR. Mini mental state: a practical method for grading the cognitive state of patients for the clinician. *J Psychiatr Res* 1975; **12**: 189–98.

4. Psychiatric symptoms in physical illness

Stroke
Parkinson's disease
Cardiovascular disease
Diabetes
Arthritis
Infection

Psychiatric and psychological symptoms in the setting of physical morbidity can have a significant impact on the management and overall outcome of the illness. Stroke comorbidity is especially common in older people.

Stroke

Depression is common in the aftermath of a stroke, occurring in up to 70% of stroke patients. The incidence peaks at about 1 month after the stroke, but the increased risk persists for at least 2 years. It is therefore important to screen for depression at regular intervals during this period. Screening may involve a standardized instrument, eg the geriatric depression scale, or it may consist of informal enquiry with the patient, and possibly the carer, into the symptoms of depression.

Depressive symptoms may be an understandable reaction to the functional impairment and associated disability of stroke. Nonetheless, if the symptoms are of sufficient severity and duration to affect recovery, a trial of antidepressants should be considered. This should be part of a more comprehensive approach involving education, occupational therapy, physiotherapy and practical support to enable the patient to cope with their physical disability.

> Just because depression appears to be 'understandable' in certain circumstances, it does not necessarily mean that treatment is not required

Depression may be difficult to separate from emotional lability (eg sudden crying episodes over trivial matters), which is often associated with cerebrovascular disease. Emotional lability may improve with the use of antidepressants, such as sertraline or trazodone.

There is some evidence that depression is more common after right-hemisphere stroke or anterior stroke, and that the risk increases with age. However, functional disability due to loss of power in an upper or lower limb is more important than whether it is a right or left hemisphere stroke.

Stroke may also be associated with pathological emotional indifference (anosdiaphosia) or denial of handicap (anosognosia), both of which can have a detrimental effect on the course of rehabilitation. When stroke is associated with receptive or expressive aphasia, it can frustrate the patient and doctor during communication, making diagnosis of the underlying depression difficult. Depression may then present as irritability, agitation, aggression or refusal to comply with rehabilitation. Cognitive deficits related to stroke may become more prominent once the focus has shifted from the physical disability. In some cases, such deficits may become global (affecting the whole brain), leading to post-stroke dementia.

Parkinson's disease

The diagnosis of Parkinson's disease often suggests that there will be a chronic deteriorating course in the patient's condition, with an increasing loss of independence. In this sense, the common occurrence of depressive symptoms and depression in Parkinson's disease is understandable. Depression continues to be underdiagnosed and undertreated in Parkinson's disease. It may be difficult to differentiate the two as they share many common features. Mask-like facies in Parkinson's disease may produce an expression simulating sadness, and the psychomotor retardation of depression may be incorrectly assumed to be part of Parkinson's disease.

There are no specific methods to differentiate depression from Parkinson's disease. However, symptoms of Parkinson's disease may vary depending on the timing of antiparkinsonian medications, eg mask-like facies or slowness may improve when the blood levels of antiparkinsonian medications are at their peak. In depression, one would not expect such dose-dependent variation.

> Depression and Parkinson's disease have many features in common, so it can be difficult to distinguish depressive symptoms in people with Parkinson's disease

Psychotic symptoms, especially visual hallucinations, are another problem in Parkinson's disease. Visual hallucinations may be the result of antiparkinsonian medications, such as levodopa, and may respond to a change in the drug regime. This can be achieved by reducing the dose or by using a slow-release preparation. A careful balance may need to be struck between controlling hallucinations by reducing antiparkinsonian medications and worsening other features of the disease. Alternatively, a small dose of antipsychotic medication could be added to the current regime. To avoid the extrapyramidal side-effects of conventional antipsychotics, atypical antipsychotics are the preferred option, for example:

- olanzapine (2.5 mg daily)
- risperidone (0.25 mg twice daily)
- quetiapine (25 mg/day, increasing to 100–200 mg/day).

Before starting antipsychotic medication, it is important to consider the frequency, severity and nature of any hallucinations, and particularly any distress associated with them. Occasionally, hallucinations may be infrequent and nondistressing, and the patient may learn to ignore them. This may be a preferred option in some patients after weighing the risks and benefits of antipsychotic medication.

> If the hallucinatory side-effects of antiparkinsonian drugs are infrequent, then antipsychotics may not be needed

Lastly, one must always be aware of the patient developing Lewy body dementia (LBD), which is more common in Parkinson's disease than was once thought. People with LBD are particularly sensitive to neuroleptics; therefore, consider giving anticholinesterases or clomethiazole (1–3 capsules/day) as a mild tranquilizer to reduce the subjective distress associated with hallucinations.

Cardiovascular disease

Cardiovascular diseases and their treatments can affect the mental wellbeing of elderly people in a number of ways. Heart attack and angina can be life-threatening experiences, as the patient starts to worry about when and where they may have another attack, and whether it will be fatal. This can lead to a preoccupation with physical symptoms, such as breathlessness, palpitations and sweating. These symptoms are also common features of anxiety, and it can be difficult to separate the two without specialist input and investigations, eg electrocardiogram (ECG). Heightened awareness of physiological functions, such as breathing and heartbeats, can lead to anticipatory anxiety about impending heart attack, further worsening of palpitations and breathlessness, and possibly a full-blown panic attack. The fear of not being able to get assistance if anything should happen to them may then lead to anxiety about going out, eventually resulting in agoraphobia.

Shortness of breath associated with congestive cardiac failure may lead to serious restriction of physical activity, affecting the quality of life and ultimately leading to anxiety and/or depression.

Coronary heart disease and atrial fibrillation are associated with an increased risk of stroke and dementia. Hypertension in middle life also leads to an increased risk of dementia, with odds ratios of 4.8 with systolic blood pressure over 160 mmHg and 4.3 with diastolic blood pressure over 95 mmHg. High levels of cholesterol, especially low-density lipoprotein cholesterol, increase the risk of developing hypertension, coronary heart disease and stroke, thus increasing the risk of dementia.

> Congestive heart failure can impose serious restrictions on physical activity, which may affect the quality of life and ultimately lead to depression

The treatment of hypertension is not without risk. Certain drugs, including propranolol, can precipitate or worsen depression by noradrenergic blockade. Antidepressants (especially tricyclics) and antipsychotics can cause cardiac arrhythmias, especially a prolonged QTc interval. Therefore the patient should be monitored for arrhythmias during tricyclic or antipsychotic therapy.

> Certain antipsychotic drugs and antidepressants can cause cardiac arrhythmias

Diabetes

Diabetes is a risk factor for both Alzheimer's disease (relative risk 1.8) and vascular dementia (relative risk 2.3). In addition, the presence of dementia may affect the control of diabetes due to the patient's inability to remember the time and dose of medications. Depression can affect appetite and also the motivation to comply with antidiabetic medications, resulting in poor control of blood

sugar levels. Hypoglycaemia is associated with symptoms such as tachycardia, sweating and dizziness, which may be mistaken for anxiety symptoms. Severe hypoglycaemia can lead to confusion. It is therefore important to rule out intermittent hypoglycaemia in patients presenting with anxiety attacks or confusion.

Arthritis

Depression is common in arthritis and may be due to chronic pain and disability; however, adequate control of the pain can prevent and treat reactive depression. Depression may also occur as a result of definitive treatment for arthritis being delayed or cancelled repeatedly, eg hip replacement operations.

Corticosteroids, sometimes used in the treatment of arthritis, are known to be associated with psychiatric problems, such as psychosis and depression.

> The chronic pain of arthritis can lead to depression

It is important to remember that painkillers, often prescribed in arthritis, are the drugs used most commonly in overdose.

Infection

Chest and urinary infections are among the most common causes of delirium, and sudden worsening in a patient with known dementia may be a result of untreated infection. The precise mechanism is not known, but it may involve increased permeability of the blood–brain barrier to toxins.

> Chest and urinary infections are common causes of delirium

Viral infections are especially important – there is no specific effective medicine and there are usually no identifiable physical signs. As a result, elderly patients may not receive adequate support. Recovery from viral infection can be a major struggle due to associated weakness and lethargy and can sometimes precipitate depression.

Further reading

Burns E, Russell E, Stratton-Powell P *et al.* Sertraline in stroke-associated lability of mood. *Int J Geriatr Psychiatry* 1999; **14**: 681–5.

Cummings J, Masterman DL. Depression in patients with Parkinson's disease. *Int J Geriatr Psychiatry* 1999; **14**: 711–18.

Launer LJ, Ross GW, Petrovitch H *et al.* Midlife blood pressure and dementia: the Honolulu–Asia aging study. *Neurobiol Aging* 2000; **21**: 49–55.

Notkola IL, Sulkava R, Pekkanen J *et al.* Serum total cholesterol, apolipoprotein E epsilon 4 allele, and Alzheimer's disease. *Neuroepidemiology* 1998; **17**: 14–20.

Peila R, Rodriguez BL, Launer LJ. Type 2 diabetes, APOE gene, and the risk for dementia and related pathologies: the Honolulu–Asia Aging Study. *Diabetes* 2002; **51**: 1256–62.

5. The multidisciplinary team

Consultant psychiatrist for the elderly
Community psychiatric nurses
Specialist social workers
Psychologists
Occupational therapists
Physiotherapists
Other disciplines
Voluntary organizations

Many specialties of medicine incorporate the multidisciplinary team (MDT) into routine working practice to provide patients with a seamless service to meet their needs. The National Service Framework for Mental Health and the National Service Framework for Older People have highlighted the need for the MDT to be the focus in delivering care to patients with mental health needs. The care programme approach (CPA) is the process by which needs are identified and care plans provided. A care coordinator is chosen from the MDT to ensure that the CPA occurs and that care is implemented and renewed regularly. The care coordinator can be any member of the MDT, depending on the initial assessment. Liaison between the MDT, GPs, district nurses and health visitors should be encouraged.

> The multidisciplinary team encompasses people from many specialties and is important in providing care for mentally ill patients

Professionals who make up the MDT in an old-age psychiatry service vary between departments, depending on local policy, resources and staffing levels. Professionals commonly found in MDT teams in the UK are discussed below.

Consultant psychiatrist for the elderly

The consultant mainly provides medical advice. This would include taking the history, performing a mental state examination, arranging a physical examination and any other appropriate investigations. Assessments will include making a diagnosis, starting treatment if appropriate, identifying risks and liaising with other members of the MDT. Some departments have the benefit of other grades of doctors, such as specialist registrars, senior house officers and staff-grade physicians.

Community psychiatric nurses

Ideally, the MDT should incorporate trained nursing staff of different grades who have experience of treating patients with a variety of psychiatric illnesses. Community psychiatric nurses (CPNs) are often identified as care coordinators within the CPA process, and also focus on educational activities, particularly for carers.

> The coordinator of a patient's care plan is often a community psychiatric nurse

Specialist social workers

In some parts of the country, specialist social workers with expertise in working with elderly mentally ill patients are very much a part of the MDT. In other areas, social work input is not integrated particularly well, and referrals have to be made to generic (nonspecialist) teams. Specialist social workers often have the added advantage of training in mental health problems and being approved under the Mental Health Act. They can not only provide assessments and provision of social care, but also have expertise in using the Mental Health Act.

Psychologists

Psychology input can be vital in several ways. Neuropsychological testing can benefit the consultants in identifying localizing symptoms. Psychological therapies such as cognitive behaviour therapy, anxiety-management training and psychodynamic intervention can assist in treatment protocols. Psychology input can sometimes be very helpful for the team itself.

Occupational therapists

It is vital to assess a patient's ability to cope with activities of daily living, to ensure that they are capable of performing both simple and complex activities, with special reference to their safety. An occupational therapist can provide an invaluable assessment before a care plan is formulated. Ideally the assessment should be carried out in the patient's home. Such an assessment can give important information about a patient's functioning and their ability to manage at home, and any necessary aids or adaptations can be put in place.

Physiotherapists

Many elderly patients have coexisting physical and psychiatric needs, and there are often complex interacting relationships between illnesses. Poor mobility can lead to a lack of independence, impaired safety and social withdrawal. By improving mobility, physiotherapy can therefore enhance independence.

> Physiotherapy can improve mobility, enhance independence and therefore relieve some of the symptoms of depression

Other disciplines

There are members of other disciplines, who, although they may not be core members of the MDT, should provide easily accessible services when needed. These may include:

- Speech and language therapists – patients often have speech difficulties, which should be identified early to aid communication. Swallowing problems are common in people with dementia; assessment and treatment, if necessary, can therefore be useful in preventing aspiration and pneumonia.

- Chiropodist (podiatrist) – many elderly patients have significant pedal problems, such as corns and ingrowing toenails. This is due to neglect, poor circulation or diabetes.

- Pharmacist – there is evidence that polydrug use is common and often inappropriate in the elderly. Pharmacists may be more aware than other members of the MDT of drug interactions, and their advice and reviews can be invaluable.

Voluntary organizations

The MDT needs to liaise closely with the relevant voluntary organizations. These offer a variety of services and can be an invaluable support to patients and carers. All professionals need to be aware of confidentiality issues when liaising with voluntary organizations.

> It is important for the multidisciplinary team to maintain patient confidentiality when working with voluntary organizations

Alzheimer's Society

The Alzheimer's Society has branches throughout the UK. It publishes leaflets on Alzheimer's disease that are easy to understand. These leaflets are available in a number of languages. The society offers support to carers, funds charitable events and is actively involved in promoting research.

Age Concern

Age Concern publishes leaflets on a variety of issues relating to elderly people, eg incontinence. It provides day-centre facilities for elderly people with or without mental illness. Individual branches may vary with regard to the range of services they provide, but examples are bereavement counselling, financial advice, advice on care and day-centre facilities.

Further reading

Lindesay J, Briggs K, Lawes M *et al.* The Domus philosophy: a comparative evaluation of residential care for the demented elderly. In: Murphy E, Alexopoulos G (eds). *Geriatric psychiatry: key research topics for clinicians.* Chichester: John Wiley, 1995: 259–73.

Ritchie K, Colvez A, Ankri J *et al.* Evaluation of long term care for dementing elderly: a comparative study. In: Murphy E, Alexopoulos G (eds). *Geriatric psychiatry: key research topics for clinicians.* Chichester: John Wiley, 1995: 275–88.

6. Legal and ethical issues

Mental Health Act
Mental capacity
Testamentary capacity
Power of attorney
Court of Protection
Advance directives
Older people and driving
Informed consent

Mental Health Act

Both GPs and hospital doctors may well encounter issues relating to the Mental Health Act during their clinical practice; a working knowledge of the Mental Health Act of 1983 is therefore important. In practice, old-age psychiatrists will always be involved where implementation of the Mental Health Act is being considered. The main purpose of the Mental Health Act is to protect the rights of people with mental illness and to enable them to receive appropriate care and treatment.

Use of the Mental Health Act should be considered when a patient appears to be or is known to be suffering from a mental illness and that patient needs assessment and/or treatment because they are a risk to themselves (through self-harm or neglect) or others (directly or indirectly), or because they are in need of treatment to prevent deterioration in their mental health, which may lead to such risks.

> The aim of the Mental Health Act is to protect the rights of mentally ill people and to ensure they receive appropriate care

Table 6.1 details the sections of the Mental Health Act, while Table 6.2 indicates those

sections that are most appropriate for certain groups of patients.

When use of the Mental Health Act is not appropriate

The Mental Health Act cannot be used to enforce treatment of physical illness, such as when a patient refuses investigation or surgery. When a physical illness is regarded unequivocally to be the cause of the mental health problem, treatment of the underlying illness may be considered in certain circumstances. Likewise, the Mental Health Act cannot be implemented for patients where there is no evidence of a mental illness, and it cannot be used for people solely with drug or alcohol dependence, especially in the case of acute intoxication.

> The Mental Health Act cannot be implemented in a person suffering only from acute drug or alcohol intoxication

Other sections

An approved social worker (ASW) can apply to a magistrate for a warrant to place a person thought to be suffering from a mental disorder and at risk of neglect by themselves or others (see Mental Health Act Section 135) in a safe environment. Similarly, any police officer can remove to a place of safety a mentally disordered person who is found in a public place and thought to be in immediate need of care, or at risk to themselves or others (see Mental Health Act Section 136). It is important to know the 'place of safety' in your area/hospital, as it varies depending on local agreements; it may be a specific ward, room, accident and emergency department or police station. The patient can be kept in the place of safety for up to 72 hours until they are assessed by a doctor and an ASW. The three possible outcomes are:

- discharge
- informed admission
- formal admission under Section 2 or 3 of the Mental Health Act.

Table 6.1
Sections of the Mental Health Act

Section	Details
2	Compulsory admission to hospital for assessment, or for assessment followed by treatment. *Medical recommendation:* two doctors, one of whom is approved under Section 12 *Application:* ASW or nearest relative *Maximum duration:* 28 days
4	Emergency admission to hospital when the requirements of Section 2 (two doctors, one approved) are likely to cause unacceptable delay, putting the patient and/or others at increased risk. *Medical recommendation:* any doctor *Application:* ASW or nearest relative *Maximum duration:* 72 hours Patient should be assessed for Section 2 by a Section 12-approved doctor as soon as possible.
5(2)*	Emergency detention of patient already in the hospital until assessment for Section 2 can be completed. *Medical recommendation:* RMO or doctor nominated by RMO (eg SHO/registrar/SpR) *Maximum duration:* 72 hours *Procedures for Section 2 assessment should be started as soon as possible.
5(4)	Emergency holding power to prevent patient with a mental disorder from leaving the ward if a doctor is unavailable for immediate completion of Section 5(2). *Application:* registered mental nurse or registered nurse for mentally subnormal *Maximum duration:* 6 hours Patient should be assessed for Section 5(2) as soon as possible. The holding order applies only when a patient is already under treatment for a mental disorder. Once Section 5(2) is completed, it lasts for 72 hours from the original time of starting Section 5(4).
3†	Admission or detention of patient known to suffer from a mental disorder for the treatment of that mental disorder, when treatment in a less restrictive environment is inappropriate because of the risks involved to the patient or others. *Application:* ASW or nearest relative *Maximum duration:* 6 months †A patient admitted under Section 3 should not be allowed to leave the ward without prior consultant approval (Section 17 form).
7	Reception into guardianship may be more appropriate for long-term treatment of patients living in the community. The guardian is usually the social services department, and has the power to require the patient to live in a particular place, attend appointments for treatment and provide access to healthcare professionals visiting the patient. *Application:* medical recommendation and duration are the same as for Section 3

ASW, approved social worker; RMO, responsible medical officer; SHO, senior house officer; SpR, specialist registrar

Table 6.2
Choice of Mental Health Act sections

Patient group	Sections
Community or A&E	
for assessment	2, 4, 25
for treatment	3, 7
for removal to place of safety	135 when the patient is at home 136 when the patient is in a public place
Already in hospital	
for assessment	5(4), 5(2), 4, 2
for treatment	3, 7

A&E, accident and emergency department

Mental capacity

Mental capacity is not universal. It relates to the situation at hand, such that a lack of capacity in respect of one situation (eg managing finances) does not necessarily mean a lack of capacity in another situation (eg choosing treatment). Capacity is also changeable: a person who does not have the capacity to manage his or her finances during a manic episode may regain that capacity after recovery from the episode.

> Lack of mental capacity in one situation must not imply lack of capacity in another situation

The Law Commission suggested that a person should be considered to be lacking mental capacity if, at the material time, he or she is unable:

- by reason of mental disability to make a decision for themselves on the matter in question
- to communicate the decision on that matter because they are unconscious or for any other reason.

There are several legal tests or criteria of capacity relating to different types of decision making, such as testamentary capacity, capacity to manage finance, capacity to enter a contract and consent to treatment and research:

- Presumption of capacity – an adult is considered to have full mental capacity until proved otherwise.
- Decision-specific capacity – capacity should be assessed separately for specific decisions.
- The doctor assessing capacity should consider the necessity (eg how necessary is the intervention?) that he or she has 'duty of care' and the patient's best interests.
- Proof – the burden of proof rests with the person assessing capacity. The standard of proof is based on civil law (balance of probability) not criminal law (beyond reasonable doubt).

- The diagnosis (eg Alzheimer's disease) does not equate to disability or lack of capacity.
- Every attempt should be made to maximize capacity, eg treat the underlying depression when a depressed person seems to lack the capacity to make decisions about the treatment of his or her physical illness, or help a patient with expressive aphasia in nonverbal communication of their decision.
- The final decision about capacity rests with the court.

Testamentary capacity

Testamentary capacity is the capacity to make a will with possession of a sound, disposing mind. A medical report is not essential, but the court may ask for a medical opinion if a will is to be contested on the grounds of impaired testamentary capacity. To have testamentary capacity, a person should:

- know that they are making a will
- understand the nature and extent of their property
- be aware of people to whom they may leave possessions
- be free from delusions that could affect their judgement in relation to the will
- not be abnormally suggestible or under the influence of drugs or alcohol.

Power of attorney

Power of attorney is usually drawn up by a solicitor. It allows a person to hand over control of their property and financial affairs to someone else. The conditions are similar to those for testamentary capacity. The person has to be of sound mind at the time of making the will. They have to have the capacity to give the power, but they may or may not have the capacity to manage all of their affairs. If they lack the latter, they need to be aware that enduring power of attorney will immediately be registered with the Court of Protection, giving someone else control of their affairs. Power of attorney lapses automatically if the person giving it (ie the patient) is no longer of sound mind. However, one can set up an enduring power of attorney, whereby the arrangements under the power persist if the person becomes mentally incapable of managing their affairs. When that happens, the power has to be registered with the Court of Protection.

> Power of attorney for a patient lapses if the patient becomes of unsound mind

Court of Protection

The Court of Protection is presided over by a Judge of the Supreme Court nominated by the Lord Chancellor. An application can be made by any interested person and can be contested by any other person. It ensures security of property and affairs, maintenance of the patient and their family. For the application to be successful, the patient must be suffering from a mental disorder and lack the capacity to manage their property and affairs. A registered medical practitioner (not necessarily a psychiatrist or a Section 12-approved doctor) has to certify the nature and effects of the mental disorder, and the patient should be given at least 7 days notice of the hearing. The receiver may be a family member, a friend or a representative of social services; they have full power, including the disposal of assets. The receiver does not have full power over the patient's medical treatment.

Advance directives

A person of sound mind can make an advance directive (forms available from charities, post offices and newsagents) with regard to different aspects of their life, including specifying the treatment they would or would not like to receive in the future. The involvement of a solicitor is not essential but is recommended. Advance directives are becoming increasingly common, but as yet they do not have a statutory framework apart from common-law (or case law) precedents. They are useful to medical professionals, as they give an indication to the patient's interest. The doctor will need to make sure that the current circumstances match closely with those expressed in the directive. Also, the time gap between the directive and current circumstances (eg a few days versus a few years), and evidence of reconsideration of the directive by the patient on more than one occasion, are important factors. Advance directives have no legal power if a person lacks capacity or is under the remit of the Mental Health Act.

> Patients are recommended to involve a solicitor when making an advanced directive

Older people and driving

Age is not a criterion in deciding upon fitness to drive. Most road traffic accidents are not caused by elderly people. A normal driving licence (not a heavy goods vehicle licence) is valid for 3 years or until the age of 70, whichever is longer. It is the responsibility of the licence holder to inform the Driving and Vehicle Licensing Authority (DVLA) about any new disability as a result of physical or mental illness, but it is the doctor's duty to make sure that the patient understands this. The doctor may have to inform the DVLA directly if the patient is unwilling to and the doctor has serious concerns about the safety of the patient or their family or other road users. The DVLA produces regular guidelines, and further advice can be obtained from their medical advisory branch (see Useful Addresses p 55).

Informed consent

Elderly people have the same rights as younger people with respect to consent, ie to receive and refuse treatment. For the consent to be informed, the doctor has to explain to the patient why the treatment is necessary, the different options that are available, the risks and benefits involved with each option, and what may happen if the patient refuses a particular treatment. The explanations should be detailed but simple enough to suit the patient's understanding. If the person lacks the capacity to consent to treatment, then the doctor should find out about the patient's interest through discussion with relatives and enquiries about advance directives. No other person, including the next of kin, can consent to treatment or research on the patient's behalf.

> The rights of elderly people regarding consent to treatment are identical to those of younger people

There are no set precedents in the law, and each case is considered independently of any previous rulings. In emergency settings, under common law, certain forms of treatment are lawful in the absence of consent if they are necessary and in the patient's best interests. For non-urgent treatment, it is useful to get a second opinion before starting legal proceedings. However, the Mental Health Act does not cover treatments for physical illnesses except in very special circumstances, ie if treatment of the physical illness is mandatory in treating mental illness, or if the physical illness is a direct result of mental illness.

> Generally, the Mental Health Act cannot be used to enforce treatment of physical illness

Further reading

Lush D. Managing the financial affairs of mentally incapacitated persons in the UK and Ireland. In: Jacoby R, Oppenheimer C (eds). *Psychiatry in the elderly*. Oxford: Oxford University Press, 1991: 951–65.

Posener HD, Jacoby R. Testamentary capacity. In: Jacoby R, Oppenheimer C (eds). *Psychiatry in the elderly, 3rd edn*. Oxford: Oxford University Press, 2002: 933–40.

7. Case studies

Case 1: depression
Case 2: confusional state
Case 3: consent in a person with cognitive impairment
Case 4: atypical depression
Case 5: dementia

In this chapter, a series of case studies, followed by comments on management, are described. These cases represent an amalgamation of clinical experience and do not refer to real patients.

Case 1: depression

A 78-year-old man was an in-patient on an acute medical ward. He had been admitted 10 days previously with weight loss of about one stone over the preceding 6 weeks and dull epigastric pain. Investigations by his GP had revealed mild anaemia and an erythrocyte sedimentation rate (ESR) of 70. He had become increasingly frail and malnourished at home. Further investigations had confirmed the mild anaemia and high ESR, and there was also evidence of significant dehydration, which was being treated with intravenous fluids.

The nurses had noticed that the patient seemed very withdrawn and did not say very much. He was always very polite when approached by the nurses, but he mainly kept himself to himself. The house officer on the ward decided to speak to him at more length about what he was thinking, and arranged to see him in a side room by himself.

The patient said that the pain in his abdomen had been getting him down for about

3 months. He felt dispirited, had lost enjoyment in his life, felt tired all the time and felt his memory was deteriorating. His family had also said that he had become more irritable. The house officer asked the patient about his personal history, and he gave the impression of a very negative view of his life: lost opportunities, dissatisfaction at work and, at times, an unhappy marriage. His wife had died 18 months previously; he found her on the floor at home after she died suddenly of a heart attack. The patient said that when he thought of his wife, he cried sometimes – they had met when they were 14 years old and got married against both their parents' wishes, when they were 17. He said that sometimes he felt that life was not worth living, and occasionally when crossing the road he had fleeting ideas of walking out in front of a car. He said that if he was run over, or he did not wake up in the morning, he would not be sad.

On testing his cognitive function, the patient scored 27/30 on the mini-mental state examination (MMSE) and 11/15 on the geriatric depression scale.

Comment

It is common to see an older person with a mixture of physical and mental health problems. The man clearly had enough symptoms to merit a diagnosis of depression, which would benefit from treatment. In addition, he turned out to have a gastric carcinoma that was inoperable. In his mental state, it was interesting to note the passive suicidal ideation that he expressed. It is very common to have symptoms of depression following a bereavement. The pervasive change of mood is indicated by his negative view of many things that went on in his life. In this situation, treatment with an antidepressant such as a selective serotonin reuptake inhibitor (SSRI) would be entirely appropriate. An alternative drug would be a tricyclic antidepressant, such as amitriptyline, which is said to be marginally more effective than SSRIs in the treatment of depression associated with physical illness; however, there are more side-effects associated with the tricyclics.

The prognosis of this situation is dependent on that of the underlying physical illness. Alerting the hospital staff to the presence of depression is likely to ensure a much more sympathetic view of the patient, rather than just someone who has chosen to isolate himself.

The opportunity for the patient to talk about his wife will probably be of benefit, but there is nothing to suggest the presence of an abnormal grief reaction. Unusual grief reactions would probably be indicated by a prolonged and obvious period of mourning associated with visions of the dead person and subjective sensations of their presence.

Case 2: confusional state

A 68-year-old man was admitted with a chest infection. After being in the ward for 2 days, he suddenly became acutely disturbed. He was aggressive to all members of the staff and seemed fearful. He appeared to be having visual hallucinations and spoke of snakes and spiders on the wall. His behaviour varied throughout the day: at times he was very quiet and appropriate, then later in the same nursing shift he would become very aggressive. He had a raised temperature, and his chest X-ray showed right middle lobe pneumonia. His blood gases showed evidence of hypoxia. The nurses requested sedation for the patient, as they had become frightened of looking after him.

Comment

This patient appears to be suffering from a confusional state but in the presence of an identifiable physical illness with two contributing factors – probable septicaemia and hypoxia. The visual hallucinations and variation in behaviour are important for the diagnosis. The presence of delirium is an acute medical emergency and demands treatment of the underlying condition. However, in a patient who becomes disturbed a couple of days after

being in hospital, withdrawal of alcohol should be considered as a possible precipitant.

In view of the patient's chest problem, one would need to be very careful about prescribing a sedative as such drugs may suppress respiration and possibly lead to respiratory arrest or, at the very least, exacerbate coexisting hypoxia. If sedative medication is required, a suitable drug would be clomethiazole 1–2 capsules up to three times daily (5–10 ml liquid up to three times daily). It is best to avoid benzodiazepines as they may also suppress respiration. If there is any doubt that delirium tremens (due to alcohol withdrawal) is a possible diagnosis, then treatment with thiamine is appropriate.

Nursing a patient with delirium includes looking after them in a well-lit room and, where possible, having the same nurse in attendance.

The prognosis in this situation is that of the underlying physical illness. The patient received antibiotic treatment for his chest infection and made a full recovery. He married his 22-year-old fitness instructor and was lost to follow-up.

Case 3: consent in a person with cognitive impairment

A 72-year-old woman with a diagnosis of Alzheimer's disease was admitted as an emergency case. She had a perforated duodenal ulcer and acute peritonitis was diagnosed. The surgeons wished to operate but asked the duty psychiatrist to see her to assess her ability to consent. They asked the psychiatrist to sign the consent form on her behalf as she was clearly unable to. On examination, the patient was clearly unwell. The story from her daughter was that she had been diagnosed with Alzheimer's disease 3 years ago and was currently being treated with donepezil 5 mg daily. She lived independently, but she was in need of increased social support at home. She was relatively well physically. She had been operated on a number of times previously and had always agreed readily to the surgery. An attempt to explain the nature of the procedure, its consequences, and the consequences of not having the procedure was not possible.

Comment

Because the patient had a diagnosis of Alzheimer's disease, her ability to consent was clearly in doubt. Legally, nobody can sign a consent form on behalf of someone else (except for a minor). However, it was clear that the patient was acutely ill, was likely to die if the operation had not been carried out, and had agreed previously to similar interventions. There was no evidence that she was a Jehovah's Witness. It was decided that in the best interests of the patient, the operation should go ahead; it did and she made a good recovery.

> Donepezil should be stopped before an anaesthetic and the anaesthetist should be made aware of all medication that the patient is taking

Case 4: atypical depression

An 84-year-old woman was admitted for investigation of multiple physical complaints. She complained of abdominal pain, a tingling sensation in both her feet, and a tight band around her head. She had been visiting her GP up to four times a day over the preceding 3 months with the symptoms. Her daughter was also a regular attendee at the GP's surgery, insisting that he do something about her mother's symptoms. The patient was seen as an outpatient and had an endoscopy, a computed tomography scan and an electromyogram – all had been normal.

The patient had been fit and well throughout her life, although following the birth of her daughter 38 years previously, she had had postnatal depression which had been successfully treated with antidepressants. Her husband had died 6 years before. She lived with her son until 9 months earlier when he moved out and got married.

On examination, she was agitated and irritable. She denied any symptoms of depression, but she was preoccupied with making sure that her son's marriage was a success and expressed doubts over the suitability of his new wife.

Comments

The patient clearly had a predisposition to becoming depressed and had somatized her symptoms. More detailed investigation merely increased and heightened anxieties that something had been missed. Her daughter may have been colluding with her symptoms by demanding action from the GP. Treatment was needed for depressive illness. Venlafaxine 37.5 mg daily increased to 75 mg daily after 10 days completely cured her of the physical symptoms. She stopped attending the GP's surgery, as did her daughter, and at follow-up 3 months later she was perfectly well, although she still did not have a good word to say about her daughter-in-law.

Case 5: dementia

A 77-year-old woman, known to have vascular dementia, was admitted to a geriatric ward after a fall. She was just about coping at home with input twice a day from social services carers and thrice-weekly visits from her daughter. She had started to wander, and was leaving pans on the stove to burn. She had gone out in the ice and snow to look for her dead husband and had slipped on the step. She was not taking any medication.

On the ward, she became aroused and aggressive, saying that the staff were trying to harm her. She needed to be held down on two occasions because she had become so agitated. The nurses were at the end of their tether in looking after her, and wanted her to be taken to an old-age psychiatry ward.

Comment

The first line of management is to educate the staff about managing the patient's behaviour. Consistency of approach is important, taking care to address her face on rather than coming from the side. It is also important to regularly explain to the patient what you are doing. In parallel to this, it is probably appropriate to use some form of antipsychotic medication.

Since atypical antipsychotics are preferred, risperidone 0.5 mg twice daily was prescribed with very good effect, reducing her level of agitation and allowing the nurses to manage her. After 2 weeks, the patient was discharged to a nursing home and was still taking the medication. Tragically, 3 months later the woman was eaten by a lion that had escaped from the local zoo.

8. Rating scales

Depression
Cognitive function
Behaviour problems
Other scales

In this chapter, some of the rating scales that may be of use in clinical practice are described. Their interpretation needs to be seen in the context of the clinical situation: the tests are only meant to be a guide and are not diagnostic in themselves. However, you will certainly impress the old-age psychiatrist to whom you refer the patient if you have completed one or more of the scales. Table 8.1 lists the assessment instruments that may be useful in patients with dementia.

Table 8.1
Assessment instruments that may be useful in patients with dementia

Cognitive function	Mini-mental state examination (MMSE) Clock-drawing test
Global assessment	Clinical dementia rating Global deterioration scale
Psychiatric symptoms	Cornell scale for depression in dementia Neuropsychiatric inventory (NPI)
Activities of daily living	Bristol activities of daily living scale

Depression

Geriatric depression scale

The geriatric depression scale (GDS) is a self-report scale designed to be simple to administer and not require the skills of a trained interviewer (Table 8.2). Each of the 30 questions has a yes/no answer, with the scoring dependent on

Table 8.2
Geriatric depression scale

Choose the best answer for how you felt in the past week:
1. Are you basically satisfied with your life?
2. Have you dropped many of your activities and interests?
3. Do you feel that your life is empty?
4. Do you often get bored?
5. Are you hopeful about the future?
6. Are you bothered by thoughts you can't get out of your head?
7. Are you in good spirits most of the time?
8. Are you afraid that something bad is going to happen to you?
9. Do you feel happy most of the time?
10. Do you often feel helpless?
11. Do you often get restless and fidgety?
12. Do you prefer to stay at home, rather than going out and doing new things?
13. Do you frequently worry about the future?
14. Do you feel you have more problems with memory than most?
15. Do you think it is wonderful to be alive now?
16. Do you often feel downhearted and blue?
17. Do you feel pretty worthless the way you are now?
18. Do you worry a lot about the past?
19. Do you find life very exciting?
20. Is it hard for you to get started on new projects?
21. Do you feel full of energy?
22. Do you feel that your situation is hopeless?
23. Do you think that most people are better off than you are?
24. Do you frequently get upset over little things?
25. Do you frequently feel like crying?
26. Do you have trouble concentrating?
27. Do you enjoy getting up in the morning?
28. Do you prefer to avoid social gatherings?
29. Is it easy for you to make decisions?
30. Is your mind as clear as it used to be?

Answer yes or no to each question

Score 1 for yes on: 2–4, 6, 8, 10–14, 16–18, 20, 22–26, 28
Score 1 for no on: 1, 5, 7, 9, 15, 19, 21, 27, 29, 30
0–10 = not depressed
11–20 = mild depression
21–30 = severe depression
GDS 15: 1, 2, 3, 4, 7, 8, 9, 10, 12, 14, 15, 17, 21, 22, 23 (cut-off of 5/6 indicates depression)
GDS 10: 1, 2, 3, 8, 9, 19, 14, 21, 22, 23
GDS 4: 1, 3, 8, 9 (cut-off of 1/2 indicates depression)

[Reproduced with permission from Elsevier Science, Yesavage JA *et al. J Psychiatr Res* 1983; **17**: 37–49. See also http://www.stanford.edu/people/yesavage/GDS.html]

the answer given. A sensitivity of 84% and a specificity of 95% have been documented, with a cut-off of 11/12; a cut-off of 14/15 decreased the sensitivity rate to 80% but increased the specificity to 100%. A 15-item version of the GDS has also been devised, and is probably the most common version in current use. The shortened version has a cut-off of 6/7 and correlates significantly with the parent scale. Logistic regression analysis has been used to derive a four-item version with a specificity of 88% with a cut-off of 1/2, and a sensitivity of 93% with a cut-off of 0/1. Sensitivity is how well a rating scale picks up an illness; specificity is how good a scale is at not diagnosing an illness which is not present. For the assessment of depression in older people, the GDS is the scale against which all others should be rated.

Brief assessment schedule depression cards

The brief assessment schedule depression cards (BASDEC) test is based on the brief assessment schedule, with the novel development of the patient choosing answers from a pack of cards to avoid the difficulties of questions being overheard on geriatric wards (Table 8.3). The scale is administered by an interviewer and takes 2–8 minutes to complete. The pack is made up of 21 cards printed in enlarged black print on a white background, and the cards are presented one at a time. Both the GDS and the BASDEC have been shown to perform identically well, with a sensitivity of 71% and negative predictive value of 86% against a psychiatric diagnosis, using a BASDEC cut-off score of 6/7.

Cornell scale for depression in dementia

This is used for the diagnosis of depression in patients with a dementia syndrome. The importance of diagnosing depression in the setting of dementia is self-evident in terms of improved diagnosis and recognition of a potentially treatable condition. Most other depression scales are completed with

---

Table 8.3
Brief assessment schedule depression cards

Each item in this scale is reproduced on a separate, large-print card. The instructions for administration are as follows:

1 Remove TRUE and FALSE cards from pack.
2 Shuffle pack of cards.
3 Hand the cards, one by one, to the patient.
4 Ask the patient to place the cards in one of two piles ('TRUE' or 'FALSE').
5 Any cards that cause confusion or doubt should be placed in a 'DON'T KNOW' pile (these may form a useful focal point for discussion).

The cards
I've been depressed for weeks at a time in the past
I am a nuisance to others being ill
I'm not happy at all
I seem to have lost my appetite
I have regrets about my past life
I'm kept awake by worry and unhappy thoughts
I've felt very low lately
I've seriously considered suicide
I feel anxious all the time

I feel life is hardly worth living
I feel worst at the beginning of the day
I'm too miserable to enjoy anything
I'm so lonely
I can't recall feeling happy in the past month
I suffer headaches
I'm not sleeping well
I've lost interest in things
I've cried in the past month
I've given up hope
True
False

Scoring
Each 'TRUE' card has a value of one point. Each 'DON'T KNOW' card has a value of half a point. The cards in the 'FALSE' pile do not score. The exceptions to this are the cards 'I've given up hope' and 'I've seriously considered suicide', which score two points if 'TRUE' and one point if 'DON'T KNOW'.

A patient scoring a total of seven or more points may well be suffering from a depressive disorder.

[Reproduced with permission from Adshead G *et al*. *BMJ* 1992; **305**: 397]

Table 8.4
Mini-mental state examination

Maximum score	Score	
		ORIENTATION
5	( )	What is the (year) (season) (date) (month) (day)?
5	( )	Where are we: (state) (county) (town) (hospital) (floor)?
		REGISTRATION
3	( )	Name three objects: (one second to say each). Then ask the patient all three after you have said them. Give one point for each correct answer. Then repeat them until the patient learns all three. Count trials and record. Number of trials _____
		ATTENTION AND CALCULATION
5	( )	Serial 7s. One point for each correct. Stop after five answers. If the patient refuses, spell 'world' backwards.
		RECALL
3	( )	Ask for three objects repeated above. Give one point for each correct.
		LANGUAGE
9	( )	Name a pencil; name a watch (two points). Repeat the following: 'No ifs, ands or buts' (one point). Follow a three-stage command: 'Take this paper in your right hand, fold it in half and put it on the floor' (three points). Read and obey the following: 'Close your eyes' (one point).
		Write a sentence (one point).
		Copy a design (one point).

Total score _____   Assess level of consciousness along a continuum

Alert   Drowsy   Stupor   Coma

information provided by the patient, but this is not always possible in dementia. The Cornell scale uses the combination of observed and informant-based questions.

Cognitive function

Mini-mental state examination

The mini-mental state examination (MMSE) is the most widely used test of cognitive function (Table 8.4). It tests the domains of orientation, language, writing, memory and praxis. It is scored out of 30, with a score of 23 or below suggesting the presence of some form of cognitive impairment.

Clock-drawing test

The clock-drawing test (Table 8.5) is a relatively new development in testing cognitive function. It is very easy to administer and is popular in primary care because of its simplicity. The patient is asked to draw a clock face and make it show a specific time, eg 2.45 or 1.10.

Table 8.5
Clock-drawing test

A priori criteria for evaluating clock drawings
(10 = best and 1 = worst)

10–6: Drawing of clock face with circle and numbers is generally intact

10. Hands are in correct position (ie hour hand approaching 3 o'clock).
9. Slight errors in placement of the hands.
8. More noticeable errors in the placement of hour and minute hands.
7. Placement of hands is significantly off course.
6. Inappropriate use of clock hands (ie use of digital display or circling of numbers despite repeated instructions).

5–1: Drawing of clock face with circle and numbers is not intact

5. Crowding of numbers at one end of the clock or reversal of numbers. Hands may still be present in some fashion.
4. Further distortion of number sequence. Integrity of clock face is now gone (ie numbers missing or placed at outside of the boundaries of the clock face).
3. Numbers and clock face no longer obviously connected in the drawing. Hands are not present.
2. Drawing reveals some evidence of instructions being received but only a vague representation of a clock.
1. Either no attempt or an uninterpretable effort is made.

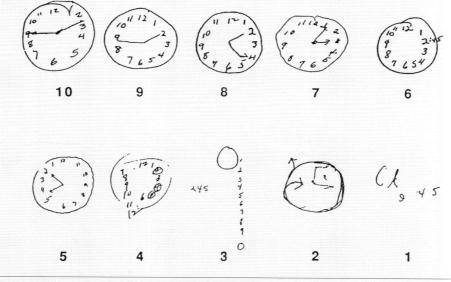

[Reproduced with permission from Brodaty H, Moore CM. *Int J Geriatr Psychiatry* 1997; **12**: 619–27]

Behaviour problems

Behavioural symptoms in Alzheimer's disease

The behavioural symptoms in Alzheimer's disease (BEHAV-AD) test is a 25-item scale that measures many of the psychiatric symptoms and behavioural disturbances associated with dementia (Table 8.6). Symptoms and disturbances are rated on a three-point scale; a second part of the scale provides a global rating of the severity of the symptoms. The BEHAV-AD is particularly useful in the assessment of patients in drug trials.

Table 8.6
Behavioural symptoms in Alzheimer's disease

Part 1: Symptomatology
Assessment Interval: Specify: _____ *weeks.*
Total Score: _____

A. Paranoid and delusional ideation
1. 'People are stealing things' delusion
0 = Not present.
1 = Delusion that people are hiding objects.
2 = Delusion that people are coming into the home and hiding objects or stealing objects.
3 = Talking and listening to people coming into the home.

2. 'One's house is not one's home' delusion
0 = Not present.
1 = Conviction that the place in which one is residing is not one's home (eg packing to go home; complaints, while at home, of 'take me home').
2 = Attempt to leave domiciliary to go home.
3 = Violence in response to attempts to forcibly restrict exit.

3. 'Spouse (or other caregiver) is an imposter' delusion
0 = Not present.
1 = Conviction that spouse (or other caregiver) is an imposter
2 = Anger towards spouse (or other caregiver) for being an imposter.
3 = Violence towards spouse (or other caregiver) for being an imposter.

4. 'Delusion of abandonment' (eg to an institution).
0 = Not present.
1 = Suspicion of caregiver plotting abandonment or institutionalization (eg on telephone).
2 = Accusation of a conspiracy to abandon or institutionalize.
3 = Accusation of impending or immediate desertion or institutionalization.

5. 'Delusion of infidelity'
0 = Not present.
1 = Conviction that spouse and/or children and/or other caregivers are unfaithful.
2 = Anger toward spouse, relative or other caregiver for infidelity.
3 = Violence towards spouse, relative or other caregiver for supposed infidelity.

6. 'Suspiciousness/paranola' (other than above)
0 = Not present.

1 = Suspicious (eg hiding objects that he/she later may be unable to locate).
2 = Paranoid (ie fixed conviction with respect to suspicions and/or anger as a result of suspicions).
3 = Violence as a result of suspicions.
Unspecified?
Describe

7. Delusions (other than above)
0 = Not present.
1 = Delusional.
2 = Verbal or emotional manifestations as a result of delusions.
3 = Physical actions or violence as a result of delusions.
Unspecified?
Describe

B. Hallucinations
8. Visual hallucinations
0 = Not present.
1 = Vague: not clearly defined.
2 = Clearly defined hallucinations of objects or persons (eg sees other people at the table).
3 = Verbal or physical actions or emotional responses to the hallucinations.

9. Auditory hallucinations
0 = Not present.
1 = Vague: not clearly defined.
2 = Clearly defined hallucinations of words or phrases.
3 = Verbal or physical actions or emotional response to the hallucinations.

10. Olfactory hallucinations
0 = Not present.
1 = Vague: not clearly defined.
2 = Clearly defined.
3 = Verbal or physical actions or emotional responses to the hallucinations.

11. Haptic hallucinations
0 = Not present.
1 = Vague: not clearly defined.
2 = Clearly defined.
3 = Verbal or physical actions or emotional responses to the hallucinations.

continued overleaf

Table 8.6 – *continued*

12. Other hallucinations
0 = Not present.
1 = Vague: not clearly defined.
2 = Clearly defined.
3 = Verbal or physical actions or emotional responses
to the hallucinations.
Unspecified?
Describe

C. Activity disturbances
13. Wandering: away from home or caregiver
0 = Not present.
1 = Somewhat, but not sufficient to necessitate
restraint.
2 = Sufficient to require restraint.
3 = Verbal or physical actions or emotional responses
to attempts to prevent wandering.

14. Purposeless activity (cognitive abulla)
0 = Not present.
1 = Repetitive, purposeless activity (eg opening and
closing purse, packing and unpacking clothing,
repeatedly putting on and removing clothing,
opening and closing drawers, insistent repeating of
demands or questions).
2 = Pacing or other purposeless activity sufficient to
require restraint.
3 = Abrasions or physical harm resulting from
purposeless activity.

15. Inappropriate activity
0 = Not present.
1 = Inappropriate activities (eg storing and hiding
objects in inappropriate places, such as throwing
clothing in wastebasket or putting empty plates in
the oven; inappropriate sexual behaviour, such as
inappropriate exposure).
2 = Present and sufficient to require restraint.
3 = Present, sufficient to require restraint and
accompanied by anger or violence when restraint is
used.

D. Aggressiveness
16. Verbal outbursts
0 = Not present.
1 = Present (including unaccustomed use of foul or
abusive language).
2 = Present and accompanied by anger.
3 = Present, accompanied by anger and clearly directed
at other persons.

17. Physical threats and/or violence
0 = Not present.
1 = Threatening behaviour.
2 = Physical violence
3 = Physical violence accompanied by vehemence.

18. Agitation (other than above)
0 = Not present.
1 = Present.
2 = Present with emotional component.
3 = Present with emotional and physical component.
Unspecified?
Describe

E. Diurnal rhythm disturbances
19. Day/night disturbance
0 = Not present.
1 = Repetitive wakenings during night.
2 = 50–75% of former sleep cycle at night.
3 = Complete disturbance of diurnal rhythm (ie less
than 50% of former sleep cycle at night).

F. Affective disturbance
20. Tearfulness
0 = Not present.
1 = Present.
2 = Present and accompanied by clear affective
component.
3 = Present and accompanied by affective and physical
component (eg wrings hands or other gestures).

21. Depressed mood: other
0 = Not present
1 = Present (eg occasional statement 'I wish I were
dead', without clear affective concomitants).
2 = Present with clear concomitants (eg thoughts of
death).
3 = Present with emotional and physical component
(eg suicide gestures).
Unspecified?
Describe

G. Anxieties and phobias
**22. Anxiety regarding upcoming events (Godot
syndrome)**
0 = Not present.
1 = Present: repeated queries and/or other activities
regarding upcoming appointments and/or events.
2 = Present and disturbing to caregivers.
3 = Present and intolerable to caregivers.

continued

Table 8.6 – *continued*

23. Other anxieties
0 = Not present.
1 = Present.
2 = Present and disturbing to caregivers.
3 = Present and intolerable to caregivers.
Unspecified?
Describe

24. Fear of being left alone
0 = Not present.
1 = Present: vocalized fear of being alone.
2 = Vocalized and sufficient to require specific action on part of caregiver.
3 = Vocalized and sufficient to require patient to be accompanied at all times.

25. Other phobias
0 = Not present.
1 = Present.

2 = Present and of sufficient magnitude to require specific action on part of caregiver.
3 = Present and sufficient to prevent patient activities.
Unspecified?
Describe

Part 2: Global rating
With respect to the above symptoms, they are of sufficient magnitude as to be:
0 = Not at all troubling to the caregiver or dangerous to the patient.
1 = Mildly troubling to the caregiver or dangerous to the patient.
2 = Moderately troubling to the caregiver or dangerous to the patient.
3 = Severely troubling or intolerable to the caregiver or dangerous to the patient.]

[Reproduced with permission from Reisberg J *et al*. *J Clin Psychiatry* 1987; **48(suppl 5)**: 9–15]

Neuropsychiatric inventory

Twelve behavioural areas are assessed in the neuropsychiatric inventory (NPI): delusions, hallucinations, agitation, depression, anxiety, euphoria, apathy, disinhibition, irritability, aberrant motor behaviour, night-time behaviours and appetite/eating disorders (Table 8.7). Each of these areas is rated on a four-point scale of frequency and a three-point scale of severity. Distress in carers is also measured.

Clinical dementia rating

This scale is used as a global measure of dementia. It is usually completed with the

Table 8.7
Neuropsychiatric inventory

Frequency is rated as:	Distress is scored as:
1. Occasionally – less than once per week.	0 – no distress
2. Often – about once per week.	1 – minimal
3. Frequently – several times a week but less than every day.	2 – mild
4. Very frequently – daily or essentially continuously present.	3 – moderate
	4 – moderately severe
	5 – very severe or extreme
Severity is rated as:	
1. Mild – produce little distress in the patient.	For each domain there are 4 scores. Frequently, severity, total (frequency × severity) and caregiver distress. The total possible score is 144 (ie a maximum of 4 in the frequency rating × 3 in the severity rating × 12 remaining domains). This relates to changes, usually over the 4 weeks before completion.
2. Moderate – more disturbing to the patient but can be redirected by the caregiver.	
3. Severe – very disturbing to the patient and difficult to redirect.	

[Reproduced with permission from Cummings J *et al*. *Neurology* 1994; **44**: 2308–14]

assessor having a detailed knowledge of the patient, as much of the information will already have been gathered as part of either normal clinical practice or a research study. If a

separate interview is carried out, about 40 minutes are needed to gather the relevant information.

Table 8.8
Confusion assessment method

Acute onset
1. Is there evidence of an acute change in mental status from the patient's baseline?

Inattention*
2. a. *Did the patient have difficulty focusing attention, eg being easily distractible or having difficulty keeping track of what was being said?*

   Not present at any time during interview.
   Present at some time during interview, but in mild form.
   Present at some time during interview, in marked form.
   Uncertain.

   b. *(If present or abnormal) did this behaviour fluctuate during the interview, ie tend to come and go or increase and decrease in severity?*

   Yes.
   No.
   Uncertain.
   Not applicable.

   c. *(If present or abnormal) please describe this behaviour:*

Disorganized thinking
3. Was the patient's thinking disorganized or incoherent, such as rambling or irrelevant conversation, unclear or illogical flow of ideas, or unpredictable switching from subject to subject?

Altered level of consciousness
4. Overall, how would you rate this patient's level of consciousness?
   Alert (normal).
   Vigilant (hyperalert, overly sensitive to environmental stimuli, startled very easily).
   Lethargic (drowsy, easily aroused).

Stupor (difficult to arouse).
Coma (unrousable).
Uncertain.

Disorientation
5. Was the patient disoriented at any time during the interview, such as thinking that he or she was somewhere other than the hospital, using the wrong bed, or misjudging the time of day?

Memory impairment
6. Did the patient demonstrate any memory problems during the interview, such as inability to remember events in the hospital or difficulty remembering instructions?

Perceptual disturbances
7. Did the patient have any evidence of perceptual disturbances, eg hallucinations, illusions or misinterpretations (such as thinking something was moving when it was not)?

Psychomotor agitation
8. Part 1.
   At any time during the interview, did the patient have an unusually increased level of motor activity, such as restlessness, picking at bedclothes, tapping fingers, or making frequent sudden changes of position?

Psychomotor retardation
8. Part 2.
   At any time during the interview, did the patient have an unusually decreased level of motor activity, such as sluggishness, staring into space, staying in one position for a long time, or moving very slowly?

Altered sleep–wake cycle
9. Did the patient have evidence of disturbance of the sleep–wake cycle, such as excessive daytime sleepiness with insomnia at night?

*The questions listed in italics under this topic are repeated for each topic where applicable

[Reproduced with permission from Inouye S *et al. Ann Intern Med* 1990; **113**: 941–8]

Other scales

Health of the nation outcome scales 65+

The health of the nation outcome scales 65+ (HoNOS 65+) is an adaptation of the equivalent scale for younger people (health of the nation outcome scale). It is a 12-item score dealing with the following aspects of the mental state and living situation:

- aggression
- self-harm
- drug and alcohol use
- cognitive problems
- physical illness and disability
- hallucinations and delusions
- depression
- other symptoms
- relationships
- activities of daily living
- residential environment
- daytime activities.

Each item is rated on a five-point scale, from 0 (no problem) to 4 (serious problem). Its main use is in the provision of the global assessment of a patient. It takes about 10 minutes to administer. HoNOS 65+ is becoming a useful tool in defining the characteristics of populations of older people with mental health problems.

Barthel index

This is probably the oldest and most widely used scale for assessing physical disability in elderly patients in general. It is often used in studies in psychiatry. Its reliability has been assessed thoroughly in four ways: by self-report, by a trained nurse and by two independent skilled observers. Agreement was generally present in over 90% of situations. Validity, reliability, sensitivity and clinical utility are all excellent. Explicit guidelines for ratings have been suggested for the scale, and an amended scoring system of 20 has been suggested.

Confusion assessment method

The confusion assessment method (CAM) consists of nine operationalized criteria from the revised *Diagnostic and Statistical Manual of Mental Disorders, 3rd edition* (DSM-IIIR), including the four cardinal features of delirium: acute onset, fluctuation in attention, disorganized thinking and altered level of consciousness (Table 8.8). Both the first and second features plus either the third or fourth feature are required for the diagnosis. The results have been validated against psychiatric diagnosis and found to be valid.

Bristol activities of daily living scale

This is used for the assessment of daily living in patients with dementia either in the community or on clinical research trials. The scale was designed specifically for use in patients with dementia and consists of 20 daily living abilities.

Further reading

Adshead F, Cody DD, Pitt B. BASDEC: a novel screening instrument for depression in elderly medical inpatients. *BMJ* 1992; **305**: 397.

Alexopoulos G, Abrams R, Young R, Shamoian C. Cornell scale for depression in dementia. *Biol Psychiatry* 1988; **23**: 271–84.

Brodaty H, Moore CM. The clock drawing test for dementia of the Alzheimer's type: a comparison of three scoring methods in a memory disorders clinic. *Int J Geriatr Psychiatry* 1997; **12**: 619–27.

Bucks RS, Ashworth CL, Wilcock GK, Siegfried K. Assessment of activities of daily living in dementia: development of the Bristol Activities of Daily Living Scale. *Age Ageing* 1996; **25**: 113–20.

Burns A, Beevor A, Lelliott P et al. Health of the Nation Outcome Scales for Elderly People (HoNOS 65+). *Br J Psychiatry* 1999; **174**: 424–7.

Burns A, Lawlor B. Craig S, Rating scales in old age psychiatry. *Br J Psychiatry* 2002; **180**: 161–7.

Cummings JL, Mega M, Gray K et al. The Neuropsychiatric Inventory: comprehensive assessment of psychopathology in dementia. *Neurology* 1994; **44**: 2308–14.

Folstein M, Folstein S, McHugh P. Mini mental state: a practical method for grading the cognitive state of patients for the clinician. *J Psychiatr Res* 1975; **12**: 189–98.

Hughes CP, Berg L, Dantziger WL *et al*. A new clinical scale for the staging of dementia. *Br J Psychiatry* 1982; **140**: 566–72 [Updated by Berg L, *Br J Psychiatry* 1984; **145**: 339].

Inouye SK, van Dyck CH, Alessi CA *et al*. Clarifying confusion: the confusion assessment method. *Ann Intern Med* 1990; **113**: 941–8.

Katona C. *Depression in old-age psychiatry*. Chichester: John Wiley, 1994.

Macdonald AJ, Mann AH, Jenkins R *et al*. An attempt to determine the impact of fourt types of care upon the elderly in London by the study of matched groups. *Psychol Med* 1982 **12**: 193–200.

Mahoney F, Barthel D. Functional evaluation: the BARTHEL index. *Md Med J* 1965; **14**: 61–5.

Novak S, Johnson J, Greenwood R. Barthel revisited: making guidelines work. *Clin Rehabil* 1996; **10**: 128–34.

Reisberg B, Ferris SH, DeLeon MJ, Crook T. The global deterioration scale for the assessment of primary degenerative dementia. *Am J Psychiatry* 1982; **139**: 1136–9.

Reisberg B, Ferris SH, Shulman E *et al*. Longitudinal course of normal aging and progressive dementia of the Alzheimer's type: a prospective study of 106 subjects over a 3.6 year mean interval. *Prog Neuropsychopharmacol Biol Psychiatry* 1986; **10**: 571–8.

Reisberg B, Borenstein J, Salob SP *et al*. Behavioural symptoms in Alzheimer's disease: phenomenology and treatment. *J Clin Psychiatry* 1987; **48(suppl 5)**: 9–15.

Sheikh JL, Yesavage J. Geriatric depression scale; recent findings in development of a shorter version. In: Brink T, ed. *Clinical gerontology: a guide to assessment and intervention*. New York: Howarth Press, 1986.

Shulman KI. Clock-drawing: is it the ideal cognitive screening test? *Int J Geriatr Psychiatry* 2000; **15**: 548–61.

Sunderland T, Hill JL, Mellow AM *et al*. Clock drawing in Alzheimer's disease. A novel measure of dementia severity. *J Am Geriatr Soc* 1989; **37**: 725–9.

Wade DT, Collin C. The Barthel ADL index: a standard measure of physical disability? *Int Disabil Stud* 1988; **10**: 64–7.

Wing JK, Beevor AS, Curtis RH *et al*. Health of the Nation Outcome Scales (HoNOS). Research and development. *Br J Psychiatry* 1998; **172**: 11–18.

Yesavage JA, Brink TL, Rose TL *et al*. Development and validation of a geriatric depression screening scale: a preliminary report. *J Psychiatr Res* 1983; **17**: 37–49.

Useful addresses

Age Concern England
Astral House
1268 London Road
London SW16 4ER
Information line: 0800 00 99 66
Web: www.ace.org.uk

Age Concern Scotland
113 Rose Street
Edinburgh EH2 3DT
Tel: 0131 220 3345

Age Concern Cymru
4th Floor
1 Cathedral Road
Cardiff CF11 9SD
Tel: 029 2037 1566

Age Concern Northern Ireland
3 Lower Crescent
Belfast BT7 1NR
Tel: 028 9024 5729

Alzheimer's Society
Gordon House
10 Greencoat Place
London SW1P 1PH
Tel: 020 7306 0606
Helpline: 0845 300 0336
Web: www.alzheimers.org.uk

Alzheimer's Scotland
Action on Dementia
22 Drumsheugh Gardens
Edinburgh EH3 7RN
Tel: 0131 243 1453
Helpline: 0808 808 3000

British Association of Occupational Therapy
106–114 Borough High Street
Southwark
London SE1 1LB
Tel: 020 7450 6480
Web: www.cot.co.uk

Carers National Association
20–25 Glasshouse Yard
London EC1A 4JT
Tel: 020 7490 8818
Carers line: 0808 808 7777
Web: www.carersuk.demon.co.uk

Counsel and Care
Twyman House
16 Bonny Street
London NW1 9PG
Tel: 020 7241 8555
Advice on residential care and benefits:
0845 300 7585
Web: www.counselandcare.org.uk
E-mail: advice@counselandcare.org.uk

Crossroads: Caring for Carers
10 Regent Place
Rugby
Warwickshire CV21 2PN
Tel: 01788 573 653

Disabled Living Foundation
380–384 Harrow Road
London W9 2HU
Tel: 020 7289 6111
Helpline: 0845 130 9177

Driver and Vehicle Licensing Agency (DVLA)
Drivers Medical Group
Longview Road
Swansea SA6 7JL
Tel: 01792 761 119
Fax: 01792 761 104

Elderly Accommodation Counsel
3rd Floor
89 Albert Embankment
London SE1 7TP
Tel: 020 7820 1343
Web: www.housingcare.org

Health Education Board
Woodburn House
Canaan Lane
Edinburgh EH10 4SG
Tel: 0131 536 5500
Web: www.hebs.scot.nhs.uk

Help the Aged
207–221 Pentonville Road
London N1 9UZ
Tel: 020 7278 1114
SeniorLine: 0808 800 6565
Web: www.helptheaged.org.uk

MIND (National Association for Mental Health)
Granta House
15–19 Broadway
London E15 4BQ
Tel: 020 8519 2122
Infoline (London): 020 8522 1728
Infoline (other areas): 08457 660 163
Publications: 020 8221 9666
Web: www.mind.org.uk

Multiple Sclerosis Society
MS National Centre
372 Edgware Road
Staples Corner
London NW2 6ND
Tel: 020 8438 0700
Helpline: 0808 800 8000
Web: www.mssociety.org.uk

National Association of Citizens Advice Bureaux
Myddleton House
115–123 Pentonville Road
London N1 9LZ
Tel: 020 7833 2181

Parkinson's Disease Society
215 Vauxhall Bridge Road
London SW1V 1EJ
Helpline: 0808 800 0303
Web: www.parkinsons.org.uk

Princess Royal Trust for Carers
142 Minories
London EC3N 1LB
Tel: 020 7480 7788
Web: www.carers.org
E-mail: info@carers.org

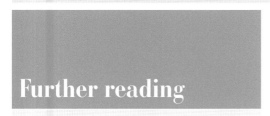

Further reading

Ames D, Chiu E (eds). *Neuroimaging of psychiatry in later life*. Oxford: Oxford University Press, 1997.

Appleby L, Forshaw D, Amos T, Barker H (eds). *Postgraduate psychiatry: clinical and scientific foundation*. London: Arnold, 2001.

Burns A, Dening T, Lawlor B. *Clinical guidelines in old age psychiatry*. London: Martin Dunitz, 2001.

Burns A, Lawlor B, Craig S. *Assessment scales in old age psychiatry*. London: Martin Dunitz, 1999.

Burns A, Page S, Winter J. *Alzheimer's disease and memory loss explained: guide for patients and carers*. London: Altman, 2001.

Butler R, Pitt B (eds). *Seminars in old-age psychiatry*. London: Gaskell Publications, 1998.

Chiu E, Ames D (eds). *Functional psychiatric disorders of the elderly*. Cambridge: Cambridge University Press, 1994.

Copeland J, Abou-Saleh M, Blazer D. *Principles and practice of geriatric psychiatry*. Chichester: John Wiley, 2002.

Dawbarn D, Allen S (eds). *Neurobiology of Alzheimer's disease*. Oxford: Oxford University Press, 2001.

Gauthier S (ed.). *Pharmacotherapy of Alzheimer's disease*. London: Martin Dunitz, 1998.

Gregoire A (ed.). *Adult severe mental disorders*. London: Greenwich Medical Media, 2000.

Growden J, Rossor M (eds). *Blue books of practical neurology: the dementias*. Oxford: Butterworth–Heinemann, 1998.

Howard R, Rabins P, Castle D (eds). *Late onset schizophrenia*. Petersfield: Wrighton Biomedical Publishing, 1999.

Jacoby R, Oppenheimer C (eds). *Psychiatry in the elderly, 3rd edn*. Oxford: Oxford University Press, 2002.

Jones R. *Drug treatment in dementia*. Oxford: Blackwell Science, 2000.

Lishman A. *Organic psychiatry*. Oxford: Blackwell Science, 1997.

Lovestone S, Howard R. *Depression in elderly people*. London: Martin Dunitz, 1997.

Murray R, Hill P, McGovern P. *Essentials of postgraduate psychiatry*. Cambridge: Cambridge University Press, 1997.

NHS Health Promotion. *Who cares? Information and support for the carers of confused people*. London: Health Education Authority, 2000.

O'Brien J, Ames D, Burns A (eds). *Dementia, 2nd edn*. London: Arnold, 2001.

Pitt B. *Psychogeriatrics*. London: Churchill Livingstone, 1982.

Tallis R, Brocklehurst J (eds). *Textbook of geriatric medicine*. Edinburgh: Churchill Livingstone, 1998.

Wattis J, Martin C. *Practical psychiatry of old age*. London: Chapman and Hall, 1994.

Wilcock J, Lux L, Rockwood K (eds). *Manual for memory disorders*. Oxford: Oxford University Press, 1999.

Index

Page numbers in *italics* refer to information shown in tables